# HAPPY HEALTHY HORMONES

Daved Rosensweet M.D.

## HOW TO THRIVE IN MENOPAUSE

# HAPPY
# HEALTHY
# HORMONES

Daved Rosensweet M.D.

## HOW TO THRIVE
## IN MENOPAUSE

This book has been written and published to provide information and should not be used as a substitute for the recommendations of your health care professional. Because each person and medical situation are unique, the reader is urged to review this information with a qualified health professional. You should not consider the information contained in this text to represent the practice of medicine or to replace consultation with a physician or other qualified health care provider.

The Menopause Method, Inc.
Sarasota, Florida
941-366-3768
www.menopausemethod.com
drr@menopausmethod.com

The Menopause Method: A Woman's Guide to Navigating Menopause, sixth edition, 2017.

Sixth Edition 2017

ISBN: 9780999744901

Published in the United States of America

# Dedication

This book is dedicated, first and foremost, to my patients in menopause: for 24 years, woman by woman, moment by moment, molecule by molecule, you have given me what has culminated in these pages. You know who you are, and I do thank you.

Writing this dedication has turned out to be a deep and heartfelt experience for me. As I'm sure so many authors have felt, this book has been a monumental project that required a village to complete! As I sit here at my computer, writing these very last words, I find myself feeling so much gratitude for so many people. My life is blessed, and has been full of colleagues and mentors who have never stopped contributing to my ongoing medical education... it's humbling. Many of these wonderful people can be found on page 253.

To my editors, Shea Lindner and Sheree Mikulec: you were willing to go into the trenches and have put so much effort and caring into this project. Thank you.

# Table of Contents

# HAPPY
# HEALTHY
# HORMONES

Daved Rosensweet M.D.

## HOW TO THRIVE
## IN MENOPAUSE

# Chapter One

# Sarah's Story

Not so long ago, I was sitting with an old and dear friend of mine, Sarah, on my porch watching the sun begin to set. We hadn't seen each other in quite some time and so had spent the day walking on the beach and being together, remembering, rediscovering, and discovering. As we sat, watching the sun wane, we had become more and more silent. The day had been sweet, and I felt content and happy. When I looked over at Sarah, however, even in the waning light, I could tell that her brow had furrowed.

"Daved," she finally said, angrily, "I have so many questions about what it is you do."

I paused and smiled. Sarah is not a combative person. Whatever she was going to say next really mattered.

"Menopause is natural," she continued, "Why should a woman go against this process and take hormones?"

I sat bolt upright, struck by the simple brilliance of her question. Sarah was the first person to come out and say so clearly what I suspect so many women in my practice must have thought.

"And Daved. . . what about breast cancer?"

I can't tell you how much I appreciated this moment. The answers to these two questions speak to the heart of why menopause has been at the center of my career for the last 24 years.

So, let's go there. Right off the bat. I'd like to share a version of just how I answered my dear friend that night.

Hormones, in both men and women, start to decline as early as our mid-thirties. Our need for them, however, does not. It turns out that hormones are important for just about everything. We need them for bone health. We need them for brain function. We need them for muscles, arteries, and bladder. The list goes on and on. Even though most women start to lose hormones in their thirties, they just don't notice it at first. Oh, there are clues: forgetfulness, irritability, and weight gain. Women just don't know to attribute some of the changes to diminished hormones.

And then, one day, comes the cessation of menses. This is the moment we think of as the beginning of menopause. It turns out, however, that it's actually just one of the more dramatic moments in that process of hormone decline. We continue to lose hormones for the rest of our lives.

As for menopause being natural, "natural" is a hard word to define. Is osteoporosis, for instance, natural? Is needing a walker or adult diapers natural? No, they are not! My most direct statement to Sarah was, "You continue to need strong bones, walking is wonderful, underpants are much more comfortable, and. . . you never stop needing hormones. Just because your body is having a hard time producing these female hormones, doesn't mean it doesn't need them!"

As she mulled this over, we moved inside. It had become so dark that we could no longer see each other.

Now, on to her second question: breast cancer. This is the one I believe almost all women contemplate. The fullest answer is that there isn't a treatment on this planet that doesn't deserve at least a little bit of risk-to-reward exploration. Think of any ad on TV you've ever seen for any pharmaceutical product. How do they go? They all start by espousing the glorious benefits and then following it up with disclaimers that are twice as long and full of all sorts of crazy, colossal, horrible-sounding side effects! Why would anyone take any of these drugs? Not that I'm an advocate for any and all pharmaceuticals (I'm not), but the reason is that often enough the good these medications can do outweighs the harm. There are possible side effects to antibiotics, but if my granddaughter came to my office with strep throat, I'm sure going to write a prescription.

So, what does the research show about hormone replenishment? A substantial section of this book is dedicated to answering this question (including a deep dive into the medical literature). The short answer is that taking bio-identical hormones not only reduces medical risk but also changes women's lives. They sleep better (a big deal). Their moods improve and their relationships get easier. Their cognitive ability returns. . . and that's just a short list of symptoms. We haven't even begun to get to the deeper, more important stuff.

The protection these hormones provide are practically everywhere: bones, muscles, brain, skin, vagina, and bladder. Hormones protect from heart attacks. The list goes on and on. To most directly address Sarah's concern: Women on properly managed bio-identical hormone regimens have a reduced occurrence of breast cancer. Reduced!

Sarah looked a bit tired, so we started gathering her belongings for her drive back to her hotel. At her car door, she paused and then asked one last question: "Daved, am I too late to start?"

I'd hoped she would ask. "No, Sarah, you are not too late. Both my mother and my mother-in-law started taking hormones in their late eighties. Both stood and walked again after barely being able to do so. After my mother's mind started disappearing, she came back to me. For a few precious extra years, I had my mom back. It's not too late."

I tell this story because it so clearly represents all of the reasons that I dove head first into this field. Why I train doctors on how to do this work properly. Why I am so passionate about this work. There are few medical specializations where the results can be so dramatic, where they happen so quickly, and where the impact occurs on so many elements at the core of overall health.

Welcome to The Menopause Method!

*Menopause in a Nutshell* 

What many women do not realize at the beginning of menopause is that there are very significant losses that commonly accompany the decline of female hormones. The losses are gradual enough, but can be oh so severe: osteoporosis, cognitive decline, loss of energy, libido, hair, muscles, and bladder function. A colleague of mine has "nailed it": natural or unnatural, for reasons known or unknown, these losses are occurring for many women!

I am understating it when I say that we humans like our hormones, all of them. And, we don't like it when they diminish. From my experience, I conclude that many women do not like how they feel, not to mention everything else that can occur when they lose a significant amount of estrogen, progesterone, testosterone, and DHEA. On the contrary, it appears to me that women so often do like it when they restore these hormones to their body. This is only the surface: what hormone treatment can mean for the bones, muscles, brain, arteries, bladder, and vagina is immeasurable in value! Beyond the medical studies, I know this is so because so many women have told me this over the years! I heard this loud and clear when a patient came into my office for a follow-up visit, glowing and exclaiming, "Gloria got her groove back!"

I am a fan of the medical, scientific literature; the short version regarding risk is that bio-identical hormones prescribed with due diligence reduce the risk of breast cancer, heart disease, stroke, osteoporosis, muscle loss, cognitive decline, and more. In this book, you will find ample references to back this up. Here are some basic points I'd like to address at the outset:

- Estrogens should be applied externally—not taken by mouth. They should be prescribed in a transdermal form (applied to skin, or in some instances, to the mucous membranes), known as "Bi-est." Testosterone, likewise, should not be taken orally. Transdermal or transmucosal application works excellently for both of these major hormones. Progesterone and DHEA are preferred transdermally but can be given orally as well.

- Transdermal and transmucosal hormone formulations are comprised of two components: a "carrier," which is known as the "base," and the hormones that are added to the base. In fact, less than 1% of the total formulation contains hormones, and over 99% is the base. Bases, understandably, contain strong solvents to obtain a uniform dispersion (solution) of hormones throughout the container. Because these solvents are strong chemicals, I am a major fan of using an organic oils formulation for the base of all transdermal and transmucosal hormone preparations. This specific base does *not* contain any solvents. For this reason, the organic oils base plus hormones is a suspension: the bottle does require a hearty shake prior to each use.

I suggest that your goals in attaining optimal dosages *of each hormone include:*

- *Healthy vagina and healthy breasts.* It is not necessary to sustain or restore youthful vaginal tissue, yet you should have sufficient estrogen to support adequate vaginal health. This can be assessed through vaginal and bladder symptoms, self-examination, pain or difficulty with intercourse, and can also be evaluated by your health professional. It turns out that if your vagina is reasonably healthy, your estrogen dosage, based even on medical studies, is most likely to be sufficient to support your bones, your arteries, and, in most but not all cases, your brain. And it doesn't take much! Benefits derive from what amounts to lowish dosages compared to those of a younger woman.

- *Zero breast and nipple tenderness.* Your breasts and nipples should not be tender. Though you are not seeking the fullness of a 25-year-old, some fullness should be present in your personal assessment. We are a "zero breast tenderness" method.

- *Muscles, energy, and libido matter.* You will need sufficient androgens, and, most importantly, you will need these androgens to sustain the health and strength of your muscles, including the muscle that supports and holds up the bladder. Androgens include DHEA and testosterone.

- *24-hour urine hormone testing is imperative.* You won't need testing initially, but you will by the time you have titrated to symptom alleviation and, thus, arrived at what seems to be your optimal dosages. Women's individual needs, as well as their ability to absorb hormones through the skin, vary so significantly that what may seem to be a low dose can produce hormone levels on testing that are excessive, and what may seem to be a very high dose can produce test levels that are too low. *Testing is imperative.* In my opinion, 24-hour urine testing is the only complete and reliable testing available for ovarian hormones.

- *Specially trained medical professional.* Furthermore, I strongly recommend working with a physician, nurse practitioner, or prescribing compounding pharmacist that has taken on the treating of women in menopause as a special professional interest and has acquired the significant training to do so. One simple, yet not all-inclusive, method of assessing expertise in this field is whether or not a practitioner is using the 24-hour urine hormone test to evaluate hormone levels. This is an essential tool. I have mentioned the general parameters regarding a "healthy vagina" and "healthy breasts." In The Menopause Method, we go on to very specifically define what we believe is the optimal dosage range for each hormone. Though relieving symptoms while falling shy of or backing down from symptoms of excess is a very helpful approach, one can be fooled by relying solely upon how a woman feels on hormone treatment! The bottom line is the 24-hour urine hormone test values obtained during treatment, which we are very specific about and address in this book as well as in our professional training program.

That is the "short" of this story. There is a "long," and here it comes to you. I am more convinced than ever that it is essential to implement hormone restoration properly and as expertly, safely, and elegantly as possible. This book provides pathways for that purpose.

And, there is more than one path! Many options and choices exist for approaching this subject. There is no universal right choice... though there is a right and wise choice for each individual woman! You will find me emphasizing the crucial importance of individualization over and over again. My objective is for each woman to learn and be "sensing" enough so as to make informed decisions and to be an active participant in the process, based on her knowledge, preferences, risks, and intuition. She will ultimately be the one discovering her way into as safe, elegant, and optimal a program as possible, day by day.

As a "bottom line," we are talking about hormones and hormones are prescription items: this process requires the assistance of a physician, nurse practitioner, or prescribing pharmacist. So, another purpose of this book is to help you to be knowledgeable enough to choose your menopause health professional wisely, based, among other things, on their alignment with your values. Their training, skills, and experience — I promise you — will matter. If you are interested, please visit our professional training website, www.menopausemethod.com. We can help you locate a menopause health professional in your area.

For those of you who would like a "sneak preview" summary of this book, go to page 317, "This Book in a Nutshell."

I wish you all so well,

Chapter Two

# Menopause: An Introduction

Menopause can sneak up on a woman, or it can seem to "drop out of the blue." At the biological bottom line of menopause, there is a major decline and imbalance of hormones produced by the ovary. Robust ovarian hormone production first begins in the early or mid-teens, peaks in the late teens and early twenties, and gradually declines from that point on. When ovarian estrogen output declines below a certain threshold, there will not be sufficient uterine lining produced to menstruate. There is a consensus that menopause officially begins one year after a woman's last menstrual cycle. At this time, the possibility of fertility is over. One thing is for sure: by then your ovarian hormone levels are very low.

Figure 2a. Variation in Hormone Levels with Age

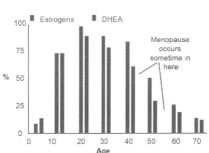

The ovarian hormones—estrogens, progesterone, and testosterone—are potent! Effects of their decline can be felt before menstrual periods cease. To give you some background on the hormone patterns in a younger woman, Figure 2b that follows is an illustration of estrogen and progesterone production during a common 28-day cycle in a regularly menstruating woman. We name "day one" the first day of menstruation. Note how estrogen levels are

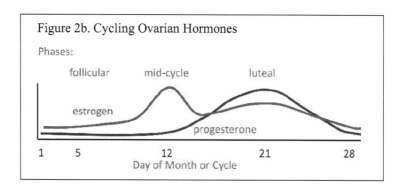

Figure 2b. Cycling Ovarian Hormones

low during days 1–5 when menstruation is taking place, rise then peak mid-cycle, decline sharply then rise again in the last two weeks, then decline to low levels. Progesterone secretion (Figure 2b) by the ovary follows a different pattern. Progesterone levels are quite low until mid-cycle. Ovulation is required for progesterone production: if (and only if) ovulation occurs, progesterone rises to robust levels. The actual rise of progesterone is better illustrated in Figure 2c below. Progesterone output can typically be +/- 30 milligrams on or about day 21, compared to 0.33 milligrams of estradiol. A woman's body sure seems to value a rich amount of progesterone! The decline of progesterone

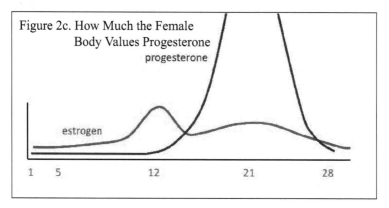

Figure 2c. How Much the Female Body Values Progesterone

production begins in the middle of the third week, then further declines by the end of the fourth week. The cascade of estrogen and progesterone to low levels at the end of the menstrual month triggers the onset of menstruation.

Alas, like it or not, over time ovarian hormone levels decline as shown in Figure 2a. Eventually, the hormone levels are so low that menstrual cycles cease altogether. As mentioned, it happens to be the level of estrogens that determine whether or not a woman will have a period. Once again, adequate estrogen levels are required for the formation of a substantial uterine lining (endometrium), and it is this lining that is menstruated. Interestingly, progesterone levels do not determine whether menstruation occurs.

When I was in medical school in the mid-1960s, we were taught the average age of cessation of ovulation coincided with the average age of the onset of menopause, which was 45 years old. Today, big differences are possible. Let's look at two situations:

- Ovulation occurring but diminished progesterone production: even if a woman is ovulating and therefore producing a substantial amount of progesterone, it is possible for her progesterone production to decline earlier and deeper than the decline of her estrogen (see Figure 2d on the following page).

- Ovulation has ceased: it is no longer necessarily so that ovulation ceases at the same time menses cease. Nowadays, it is not uncommon for ovulation to cease years before menstrual cycles cease, even as much as ten years earlier.

The consequence in both of the scenarios above is that there is relatively less progesterone and, ultimately,

Figure 2d. Earlier and More Profound Decline of Progesterone

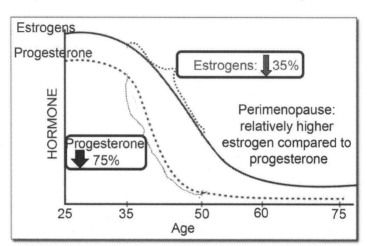

insufficient progesterone to balance the stimulatory effects of the estrogens. Again, a woman does not need to ovulate to have a menstrual cycle. And, if she does not ovulate, she can have a cycle that has disproportionately reduced amounts of progesterone.

Figure 2d above is an important illustration (thank you to Michael Lam, M.D.[2.1]) of this more-common-than-ever first possible issue: an earlier-in-life and more dramatic decline of progesterone, as compared to estrogen decline. This disproportionate decline is one of the first possible challenges that can take place during "perimenopause." It can begin a very significant imbalance: there is insufficient progesterone to balance the stimulatory effects of estrogen. At this time, symptoms can begin to appear that relate to progesterone insufficiency.

Perimenopause is the "zone" that marks the beginning of symptoms of hormonal decline—and begins the progression towards the deeper consequences of further declines.

The next, and major, event that can take place is the cessation of ovulation altogether as depicted in Figure 2e below, thus, the end of the production of any significant amount of progesterone.

Figure 2e. No Ovulation: Minimal Progesterone

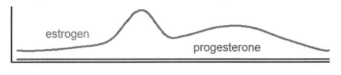

Why should there be such historical changes, both the earlier and greater decline of progesterone as well as an earlier average age of cessation of progesterone production, when ovulation ceases prior to menopause? The reasons for these two types of dramatic change are many, including increased exposures to medicinal and environmental hormones (such as birth control pills and birth control pill contamination of our water supply) along with environmental toxins that behave chemically as estrogens. In both cases, the elegant balance of hormones in a woman is disturbed, often enough beginning at young ages.

Under ordinary circumstances in young menstruating women, estrogen and progesterone are in a synergistic balance with one another. Estrogen stimulates: it stimulates breast glandular tissue in preparation for possible breast-feeding, and it stimulates the uterus to form an endometrial lining. Estrogens do have an additional function: they will even mobilize for the stress response to support "fight-or-flight." Progesterone, on the other hand, quiets. It balances estrogen. It calms the mind and aids in sleep. Progesterone rubbed on fibrocystic breasts can often "quiet down" the over-stimulation from estrogen.

Once again, the consequence of both the earlier and more rapid decline of progesterone than estrogen over time, as well as the possible earlier cessation of ovulation, results in insufficient progesterone to balance the stimulatory effects of estrogen. Thus, women who have insufficient progesterone have domination of estrogen effects and can develop increased breast density, fibrocystic breast disease, uterine fibroids, and other adverse consequences. So many hysterectomies and other issues could be averted by early detection and treatment of progesterone deficiency early in perimenopause.

Thus, it is remarkably practical for a woman and/or her health professional to be able to identify a relative progesterone decline as well as the cessation of ovulation so that progesterone treatment can be implemented. Many times, women do not think of themselves as being in perimenopause or menopause if they are still having periods. Yet, it is not difficult to identify a decline in progesterone, either the "early relative type" and/or the "abrupt type," that comes from ovulation ceasing. When an early and relative progesterone deficiency is coming on, it is common to find symptoms of "estrogen dominance" appearing. When ovulation ceases, the progesterone deficiency becomes even greater. One common manifestation of the cessation of ovulation is when a woman with a history of very regular periods begins having irregular cycles, shorter and/or longer than usual. So often, this is a sign that ovulation is not occurring, as a hallmark of regular periods is regular ovulation. Other common manifestations can occur in women who have had relatively easy periods, such as breast tenderness, PMS, and significant uterine cramps. These symptoms are caused by estrogen-induced overstimulation of the breast's glandular tissue and the uterus, which are not balanced by the calming effects of progesterone. Such phenomenal good can be done by women and practitioners who identify early progesterone decline and/or cessation of ovulation and then begin treatment with progesterone.

> ### *So much good can be done by identifying early progesterone decline, and/or loss of ovulation, and treating with progesterone*

*Symptoms and Effects of Ovarian Hormone Insufficiency*

Let's look more closely at the symptoms and effects of insufficiency of estrogen and progesterone. This will assist us in identifying the time to consider whether and when to treat with these hormones.

Again, progesterone calms. Intravenous injection of the right dose of progesterone (though never commonly done) could put anyone into a sleep so deep that surgery could be performed on them. It makes sense that common symptoms of progesterone deficiency can include a lack of calmness, such as unexpected anxiety and disturbances in the ability to sleep. Also, as I have mentioned, symptoms can develop when progesterone is no longer sufficiently present to balance estrogen. Thus, a woman will experience a dominance of estrogen stimulation—again, such as overstimulation of breast glandular tissue with breast tenderness, nipple tenderness, breast fullness, fibrocystic breast issues and breast growth, overstimulation of the uterus, PMS, heavy menstrual flow, etc.

In Figure 2f below, I summarize the symptoms of progesterone insufficiency.

Figure 2f.

PROGESTERONE

Too little:
- Sleep disturbance*
- Increased anxiety
- Mood disturbances
  (sometimes severe)
- Hot flashes*
- Breast tenderness*
- New &/or enlarged breast lumps

- Water retention*
- Difficulty relaxing
- Decreased libido*
- Period irregularities
  (if still menstruating)
- PMS, fibroids, &/or
  endometriosis

To understand estrogen deficiency, let's begin with a description of natural estrogen effects by Uzzi Reiss, M.D. The following quote is from his book *Natural Hormone Balance for Women:*

"Estrogen makes you feel sensual.
It brings glow to the skin,
moisture to the eyes,
fullness to the breasts,
and clarity to the mind.
It keeps the vagina lubricated.
It uplifts and stabilizes your mood.
It influences your brain and your bones,
and protects you against cardiovascular disease..."

Estrogen deficiency generates different types of symptoms. Some of the more common ones are the "vasomotor" mysteries of temperature swings, very familiar to any woman who has ever experienced hot flashes, warm rushes, and night sweats. When these occur in the middle of the night, they can bring forth yet another kind of sleep disturbance that is caused by a different mechanism than the sleep disturbance of inadequate progesterone. The origin is the nocturnal hot flash, and a woman can awaken either feeling the hot flash... or not. At times, she will awaken just after the hot flash, having kicked off the covers, or awaken with a nightgown wet with sweat. At other times, she will awaken and only notice her mind is "racing." There is an aspect of the hot flash that involves adrenaline secretion, which is a very energizing event! And there she lies, wide awake until her liver adequately metabolizes and eliminates the jolt of adrenaline fueling her excessive thinking. Younger people with healthier livers eliminate coffee and adrenaline much quicker than those in mid-life. Thus, that nighttime awakening often has to be endured for a longer time than desired in a woman who no longer has youthful liver power.

It is not uncommon for blood pressure and/or pulse rate to rise from the adrenaline surge, whenever it takes place. Estrogen deficiency, probably through the mechanism of adrenaline, can lead to a racing heart, palpitations, and even chest pain. It is not uncommon for a perimenopausal or menopausal woman to go to an emergency room with palpitations and chest pain fearing a heart attack. So often, even advanced testing such as an angiogram shows no signs of coronary atherosclerosis in many of these women.

Unquestionably, women can experience a variety of symptoms and effects from estrogen deficiency. Let's take a look at a few more:

- "Brain Fog," which can manifest as a range of cognitive dysfunctions from forgetfulness to slow and even significantly compromised memory and/or thinking.

- Weight Gain. Yes, estrogen deficiency can also relate to weight gain. Estrogen is an excellent stress hormone. When it declines, the body must rely even more on cortisol for the stress response. Increases in cortisol can lead to insulin resistance, and this is a recipe for weight gain, especially with simple carbohydrate dietary indiscretions.

- Osteopenia and/or Osteoporosis. There is a five-year period, from later perimenopause onward, where diminished estrogen has a particularly detrimental effect on the bones and when bone loss can be the most pronounced.

- Vaginal Dryness and Eventual Atrophy. Longstanding estrogen deficiency invariably leads to vaginal dryness and eventual atrophy. From this follows pain and difficulty with intercourse. Vaginal atrophy can also lead to irritation of the urethral opening in the vagina with ensuing bladder symptoms of urgency, frequency, and having to arise in the night to urinate — yet another sleep disrupter.

- Headaches and even Migraines. Treating women with so-called "menstrual migraines" (usually occurring one or two times per month when the estrogen levels have fallen very low) with estrogen can make such an appreciated difference.

- Coronary and Cerebral Arteriosclerosis, thus for a heart attack or stroke.

- Alzheimer's Disease. As I mentioned before, estrogen deficiency is even a risk factor for Alzheimer's disease.

In Figure 2g below, I summarize the symptoms of estrogen insufficiency. You can also find the charts on estrogen and progesterone deficiency at the end of this book.

Figure 2g.

**ESTROGENS**

Too little:

- Warm rushes
- Night sweats
- Sleep disturbance*
- Mental fogginess
  &/or forgetfulness
- Weight gain (primarily
  thighs, hips &/or buttocks)
- Dry vagina, eyes &/or skin
- Diminished sensuality
  & sexuality*
- Sense of normalcy only
  during 2nd week (if cycling)
- Hot flashes*
- Temperature swings
- Racing mind at night
- Fatigue or reduced stamina
- Episodes of rapid heartbeat
  &/or palpitations
- Pain during intercourse
- Loss of glow
- Back &/or joint pain
- Intestinal bloating
- Headaches &/or migraines

As you can see and may have experienced, progesterone and estrogen deficiency symptoms can be quite disruptive. Of more profound significance are the deeper, adverse consequences of ovarian hormonal deficiency that, over time, can affect tissues and organs.

I cover all of these subjects including numerous references to the scientific medical literature in a teaching program designed for professionals. For those of you who are interested in plumbing the scientific basis for much of what is included in this book, beyond the references in Appendix B, you can obtain it through our training program for medical professionals at www.menopausemethod.com.

The deficiencies of these hormones, the estrogens and progesterone, are at the cornerstone of perimenopause and menopause. As I stated before, often the first issues that can develop result from the earlier and deeper decline of progesterone. This decline will be followed by the cessation of regular ovulation with the attendant cessation of most all significant progesterone production. As a result, the balancing effects of progesterone are not in place and over-stimulation from estrogen will occur. And, as ovarian function continues to decline, anywhere between slowly-but-surely and precipitously, the symptoms from estrogen deficiency can arise.

Androgen deficiency, principally of testosterone and DHEA, with all of the attendant adverse consequences, sooner or later will occur in menopausal women. It may not be present initially; it may take a few years after the onset of menopause to develop. It will develop. Androgen deficiency is rife with issues including loss of muscle mass and strength, bladder support, stance and gait instability, a decline of energy, mood, and libido. We will examine androgens in more detail in a later chapter.

Many a strong woman has successfully "weathered" menopause and the commonplace insufficiency symptoms, such as hot flashes. Of more crucial importance to the women that have them are the sleep disturbances, energy losses, unwanted weight gain, mood fluctuations, and cognitive dysfunctions. These are life disrupters! Additionally, and from a medical standpoint of great significance, there are the silent but potentially problematic consequences to the mind, brain, muscles, bones, bladder, and arteries (to name a few) from the disappearance of these hormones.

As a physician, I have had the opportunity to observe the ultimate effects of hormone depletion, even to devastating proportions. I have seen elderly women in their 80s and 90s fall from the instability of weak lower extremity musculature. I've witnessed hip and other bones fracture, cognitive dysfunction — sometimes severe — and coronary artery disease. I've seen bladder problems galore. Though these are not inevitable for all women (many never develop these problems), the incidence of occurrence is high. It is super-high if it happens to you or a loved one!

Because of the consequences of hormonal decline, I am a major advocate of hormone replenishment whenever it is medically proper for a woman.... not too much, not to youthful levels, and not too little. Wonderfully, it just doesn't take that much to make a major difference.

We have also developed hormone formulations specifically for elderly women and have had successes with them. To learn more about these, please visit www.menopausemethod.com, our website for medical professionals. From the home page, click on "MM-Elder" and view the videos.

Please know, I am not here to frighten you. Yet, it is important that I present this information that is so prevalent in clinical practice and so profuse in the medical literature. As I state when I am instructing doctors:

> There may be risk in treating with hormones
> (though this is debateable):
> there is near certainty of adversity from not.

Now there's a statement! And doesn't it lead into a subject that I believe is on the mind of every woman who is considering hormone replenishment: risk? In the next chapter, I am going to delve deeper into the risks and benefits.

Menopause is a complex process. It requires time and dedication to arrive at a safe, reliable, individualized, and effective program. The ability to fashion a safe and precise menopausal strategy is more possible than ever before. I encourage you to focus on the fine points in order to engage in the discovery of your optimal program.

In light of all this complexity, it is also true that many women have a very easy time in menopause. Ultimately, this information is all about making your tailored menopausal program as safe, easy, and elegant as possible.

Chapter Three

# Risks and Benefits

## *Risk: The Bottom Line*

In 2002, a "seismic shift" took place in the world of menopause. The totally unexpected results of an extensive medical study, the Women's Health Initiative (WHI),3.1 announced a very small but statistically significant increased risk of breast cancer, heart disease, and more from "hormone replacement therapy" (HRT). The HRT used in the study were two pharmaceutical medications: Premarin® and Prempro®. Premarin consists of estrogens derived from horse urine. Prempro is a combination of Premarin plus an artificial problematic "progestin" named medroxyprogesterone acetate. To be emphasized, only the Prempro arm of the study was discontinued because of small but measurable, increased risks. The arm of the study that examined Premarin alone did not find any increased risks, and they continued that part of the study. The news of the results from this study spread like wildfire. Patients and physicians alike were impacted to the extent that many women abandoned their treatments and many physicians ceased prescribing hormones for women in menopause.

In the years that have followed the publication of the WHI, there have been several developments. First to occur were the follow-up investigations, which involved a closer examination of the WHI scientific study itself. Uncovered, were valid faults in the study design. Attempts were made to point out the problems, reinterpret, and minimize the results: to "put the cat back in the bag." It was too late. The fear of hormones and hormonal treatment had ignited and persists to this day. Of significance was another outcome: though many of the women who abandoned hormonal treatment endured the onslaught of symptoms and the attendant underlying adversities, others chose not to forgo treatment. Optional treatment methods were found and pursued by many. Treatment with bio-identical hormones, already "around" for 20 years, moved to the foreground. Even pharmaceutical manufacturers began producing their own versions of bio-identical ovarian hormones.

For many years, I have extensively investigated the science involved in risk and want to summarize my conclusions. Again, for those of you who would like to research this subject in depth, I refer you to our extensive professional training program, www.menopausemethod.com, that offers 300 references on this topic and many others related to menopause and hormones. Here are my conclusions:

- Bio-identical hormones that are properly administered do not cause cancer.

- Cancer causes are strong, deep, and multifactorial. The causes ultimately stem from a multitude of long-term issues related to nutrition, toxicity, how one responds to stress, and exercise.

- Well-differentiated, non-primitive breast cancers that have the biologic and biochemical structure and function similar to the parent breast glandular cell from which they mutated have microstructures amongst them which are estrogen and progesterone receptor sites. If you give estrogen to a woman who already has present but yet-undetectable breast cancer developing (it takes 10 to 15 years for a cancer to grow from one cell to a detectable lump), it will stimulate the growth of that pre-existing cancer — it will grow faster and become apparent sooner.[3.2]

- Medroxyprogesterone acetate, the "pro" part of Prem-pro, is problematic and *is* related to increased risk.

- Treatment with "bio-identical" estrogens and proges-terone are associated with a lessened risk of cancer, heart disease, and other medical conditions, compared to no treatment at all.[3.3] According to the WHI study, treatment with Premarin alone was also associated with less risk than no treatment.

- Hormones are potent. Prescribing them requires the utmost of training, knowledge, skill, and experience to implement in such a way that it reduces risk and increases benefits as much as possible. An overdose of any hormone will cause medical problems.

- In current times, there are practitioners who have a significant amount of knowledge and expertise that are practicing good menopause medicine. Also com-mon are the practitioners who are well-meaning but unaware of the substantial body of knowledge that exists regarding menopause and natural hormones and, in my opinion, fall shy of medical practices that overall minimize risk and maximize benefit. There are also popular menopause treatment regimens that advocate robust dosages of hormones that again, in my opinion, are not appropriate given all we currently know, as they may put women at risk.

- The "final answers" about risk are not in yet. More research on bio-identical hormones and hormone dos-age regimens needs to be done.

*Benefits*

For decades prior to the WHI, it was well known that there were many benefits to HRT. For years, Premarin had been the #1 best-selling medication in the U.S.A. So many women appreciated the symptom relief.

Many physicians have been aware that the incidence of a heart attack from coronary artery disease is greater in young men than in young women. By age 60, the incidence eventually equalizes in both genders. One significant difference was thought to be estrogen. One of the objectives of the WHI was to prove this and expand the market share for the drugs. The study design, even in this regard, was flawed; the results showed the contrary. Many other medical studies have verified the benefits of hormones for coronary arteries.[3.4]

Furthermore, the scientific medical literature makes it clear that women in menopause who are prescribed hormones have a lesser incidence of cognitive deterioration, Alzheimer's disease, colon cancer, osteoporosis, vaginal atrophy, dental loss, macular degeneration, and other seriously debilitating conditions.[3.5]

We do know that women are at risk for breast cancer. That risk has increased from 1 in 20 to 1 in 8 over the course of my medical career. There are many reasons for this increase in incidence, and these reasons need to be addressed.

Yet, studies to date do not demonstrate an increased risk when using bio-identical hormones in reasonable dosages if there is not a pre-existing breast cancer. In fact, women using bio-identical hormones have a lesser risk than women receiving no treatment at all.[3.6]

Risks from hormone depletion need not only be ascertained from the medical literature. Beyond the common, well-known menopausal symptoms, so many women experience energy loss, sleep disturbance, cognitive dysfunction, memory loss, mood deterioration, libido decline, vaginal atrophy, bladder disturbances, weakening of muscles leading to a propensity to fall and, after that fall, the fracturing of osteoporotic bones as age increases and hormones diminish. The case to replenish these hormones and experience the multitude of benefits is very strong!

In general, the risk of adverse health events does exist. I am not here to minimize this. According to the medical literature, the risk from taking hormones cannot be totally dismissed. Our knowledge of risk calls for a new level of precision and excellence in the evaluation and treatment of women in menopause. For decades prior to the WHI and even continuing today, many women have been receiving care that, in my opinion, is not excellent or even acceptable. In addition, there are many past and current practices that border on risky.

> As an example, F.S. came to me as a patient when she was 60 years old. She had been on Premarin for 20 years and was curious about the possibility of trying bio-identical hormones as she had heard "good things" about them. On detailed questioning, I heard from her that she had never had breast tenderness in her life until she went into menopause at age 40 and was prescribed Premarin. She then went on to have breast tenderness for 20 years. I am not implying that Premarin was the main problem here, only that she was on what I consider to be an excessive dose: estrogens excessive enough to overstimulate breast glandular tissue. At the very least, this was a case of

improper monitoring and dose adjustment, together with no existing method or ability to test the hormone levels of Premarin.

Increased risk also pertains to excessive dosing of other estrogen preparations.[3.7] Commonly enough, our group uncovers excessive dosage levels when we do a confirmatory 24-hour urine hormone test. Most women will feel symptoms of overdose—but not all. As part of The Menopause Method protocol, when a woman arrives at her optimal dosages clinically, we do a confirmatory 24-hour urine hormone test (and we repeat that test as a routine every 1 to 1.5 years). For its ability to test a woman while she is taking hormones and, among other things, to uncover overdose when there are no obvious symptoms of it, I am a profound advocate of 24-hour urine hormone testing.

Many women, through resilience and other factors, have done good enough on regimens based on the simple prescription of pills (with one or two doses fitting all) with little to no hormone testing and overall monitoring. However, it is the vulnerable women, for all of the reasons that vulnerability to illness exists, who are most at risk for the adversities, minor to major. Yes, because of human resilience, much can be "gotten away with." Again, for the more vulnerable this may not be so, and harm can occur.

Risk calls for excellent care. Any individual that has taken the time and effort to implement a health enhancement program realizes that commitment to education, time, energy, details, and practice is needed with respect to the subject of nutrition, exercise, toxicity reduction, and emotional healing. Similar devotion to knowledge and implementation is required for women in menopause. It is important to reverse personal negative health trends and develop approaches to recover and enhance health. Additionally, because hormone depletion is involved in the aging process for women and men, a healthcare practitioner (with a license to prescribe hormones) is required to address these deficiencies. Hormones are powerful and must be prescribed and monitored with significant expertise. In the prescription of hormones, a level of knowledge, attention to details, and precision is likewise certainly called for! The body of knowledge from which this expertise partially derives is now very substantial, and attaining it requires specialized education.

I am of the very strong opinion that the standards of training and care for health professionals in treating women in menopause should be upgraded to levels of education, certification, and expertise that prevail for other specialties in our traditional medical world. The body of knowledge in treating women in menopause has mushroomed over the past two decades. This has led to methods of evaluation, testing, and monitoring which I will specify later in this book. It is still probable for women to seek and receive care that will be fine for the resilient but potentially risky for the frail. One of my intentions for writing this book is to share with you what I believe is of crucial importance when choosing a practitioner to assist you. Another reason is to help you understand sufficient details about the process of evaluation, prescribing, and ongoing monitoring programs that rise to the level of minimizing risk and maximizing benefit with hormonal treatment. With this information, you will be able to evaluate if any proposed care is optimal for you, and you will be prepared to be an active participant in that process.

Many medical professionals involved in menopause are currently working to popularize and upgrade the training programs for physicians and nurse practitioners. I encourage you to seek assistance from excellently trained and qualified practitioners for the primary intention of bringing your personal risk as close to nil as possible while enhancing your opportunity to maximize the important benefits.

I have drilled down into the initial layer of the subject of risks and benefits because one of the very first things a woman encounters after she identifies the possibility that her hormones have declined is the choice to treat with hormones, or not. She meets up with the subject of possible risk. Her ultimate decision relies partly on her own intuition and knowledge, along with the knowledge of her medical professional and her trust in her or him. This intuition relates to the subject of risk in general as well as relating to her specific risks and benefits. I always encourage my patients to pause if they have not reached clarity after a professional consultation and review of the medical information. For example, if it is not clear what path feels right for you, treatment or no treatment, I recommend that you honor this reluctance and keep in the process until the answer becomes clear. Your instincts, along with pursuing the general and specific information will get you there. A delay before choosing will be fine. We like to avoid prescribing hormones to any woman who has trepidations about using them. For instance, we do not want a situation where every time a woman is applying hormones on her skin she has significant concern that she "could be causing cancer." Whatever the reason for her concern, it is worth pausing and honoring. With due diligence and time, the clear personal answers will emerge.

No path is "written in stone." If treatment is embarked upon, a decision to stop can occur at any time without consequences beyond those of the return to the baseline situation: symptoms and risks of diminished hormones. To be remembered is that throughout the long history of women on Earth, the vast majority of women never received treatment with hormones. That does not mean they did well, but many did quite well enough. In addition, if a decision is made to stop hormone treatment, then at some point in the future, a decision can always be made to start again.

The risk of illness does exist. This is the planet Earth, where illnesses can and do occur. Again, causes that relate to risk originate from issues of nutrition, toxicity, exercise, and stress. Causal events from these issues are many and are lifelong. And, great mysteries also still exist as to who, why, when, and so on regarding illness. As you can begin to see, the potential or actual risk from hormones has a complexity to it: there is certainly more to this subject than "meets the eye!"

*There may be risk in treating*
*with hormones, though*
*this is debateable:*
*there is near certainty*
*of adversities from not.*

Chapter Four
# General Principles of Menopause

*Individuality and Individual Variation*

As all of us know, there are significant differences, person to person, in humanity. We are unique from one another. Women are unique, and from one to another. There are similarities for sure. However, the differences are important to understand, and they have practical ramifications. For example, in medicine, so many physicians and nurse practitioners are aware that what constitutes a low dose for one person could amount to an excessive dose for another, especially for a very "sensitive" individual.

Women come in all sizes and shapes. Part of the physical differences in body types are determined by variations in hormonal levels and patterns. Practically speaking, this makes "one dose fits all" an often ineffective and mediocre treatment strategy. Excellent treatment programs are important and call for individualization of each woman and her treatment program. Individualized assessment, treatment, and monitoring programs require time and attention to detail. They also require flexibility to respond to the changes and the unexpected over time, all hallmarks of good menopause medicine. There is no way around individualization, nor should there be. It adds to the safety, excellence, and elegance for women. The complexity and variations can also keep the work constantly interesting for the medical professional.

My first vivid encounter with an important aspect of individuality came many years earlier in my career when

I was learning from a physician by the time-honored tradition of "shadowing" him in his office. As we emerged from the consultation room, Dr. Gaby spoke to me about the patient we had just examined:

"This woman is hypothyroid. To treat her, interestingly enough, you haven't a clue of what dose of thyroid hormone to write on your prescription pad. People vary so much as to the amount of hormone that they need, their ability to absorb and assimilate whatever you give them, and their individual sensitivity to whatever you prescribe. But, no worries, we'll teach her how to find her own dose."

I was startled! He had gone to medical school. I had gone to medical school. Up until that time, no one had ever taught us to have a patient "find their own dose" of anything, ever! Yet, this pioneer physician was correct. Individuality has to be respected clinically, right down to the determination of the hormonal dose in order to achieve an optimal outcome. Understanding and implementing this important approach to individualizing dose determination makes a world of difference!

We see individual differences in risk. We see variability in the often difficult-to-interpret wideness of clinical laboratory ranges. We are constantly working with patient-to-patient variabilities of absorption, idiosyncrasies, sensitivities, compliance, commitment, willingness, economics, and a host of other factors. Working with these complex variables is often part of the "art" of medicine. Being a physician requires, among other things, an interesting combination of highly precise and focused attention to detail, a great acceptance of complexity, and generous measure of loosey-goosey flexibility.

Individuality and individual variation: you will encounter it everywhere. You are an individual with your own wants, needs, risks, intuition, preferences, sensitivities, pocketbook, etc., etc. The more you know, the better equipped you'll be to assist in the fine-tuning of your overall health and menopause program. You will be able to make adjustments that best fit who you are, what you want, and what is working and not working for you.

*Beyond the Ovaries: The Knee Bone is Connected to the Thigh Bone...*

Hormones play a fundamental role in the normal day-to-day biology in our bodies. That is their principle function and importance. However, there is another role that they are capable of playing, which is in mobilizing body physiology for the biological stress response. It is this extraordinary adaptation that allows us to fight or flee from a sabre-toothed tiger. This same stress response is also quite active when we are worrying about finances, people, relationships, etc. Biologically, our bodies cannot distinguish between a tiger or a cash flow problem.

Is this a problem? Well, usually. The fight-or-flight biochemistry recruits precious adrenaline, cortisol, and insulin into the stress pathways. It also can and will call estrogens, androgens and thyroid, as well as neurotransmitter

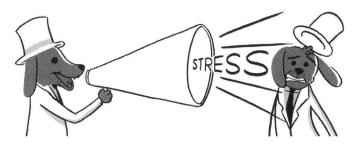

biochemicals to its service. This is not too consequential in the short run for the young of age. However, should a dysfunctional response to stress recur too frequently, it ultimately takes a toll on us physically. Though our bodies can "rise to the occasion" in the short run, over the long haul we cannot endlessly continue to keep up with the biological hormone and neurotransmitter production that comes from the excessive demands of unskilled responses to stress.

One interesting example of this relates to estrogens. Their primary function pertains to female physiology. They also will be chosen in times of amplified stress to do their part in animating for fight-or-flight. Thus, it is common among younger, stressed women (emotionally and/or physically) to have their estrogens diverted down the biological stress pathways and away from female functions. These women can often develop ovulation and period irregularities, or absence.

With chronic, dysfunctional responses to stress, we ultimately develop depletions and imbalances of hormones and neurotransmitters, among other things. This plays into the treatment of menopause. If there has been excessive stress over extended periods of time, hormone deficiencies and imbalances will be more pronounced than what would simply be attributable to menopause. There can also be long-term deleterious effects on other systems that are best taken into account and addressed at this time.

Also, if there is variability in ongoing stress responses, there can be variations and irregularities in the dosages required in treating women in menopause. Additional and challenging-to-predict hormone treatment is intermittently needed to supplement the recruitment of hormones by the stress response. Maintaining an "even keel" hormonally during periods of stress can be a challenge.

I would like to emphasize that it is not the stress per se that is the problem. This is Earth. We are human, and life on Earth is rather "loaded" with stress. It is unlikely that stress will be eliminated in our lifetime. Nor does it need to be. It is not the stress we encounter that is the main health issue—it's how we respond to it. Are we calm, cool, collected, and compassionate, or do we "flip out" inside and out? The latter response brings with it the cascade of hormones and biochemicals of the biological stress response, along with the short and long-term consequences. The ability to meet and respond to stress in a skilled and successful way, without the triggering of one's internal biology of the stress response, is a great gift to ourselves and the world.

This is a grand and wonderful topic and, these days, an enormous amount of information and support is available from a tremendous number of resources. I also extensively address this subject elsewhere (www.iwonderdoctor.com) in detail. It is all about information, tools, support, and a personal healing practice related to the emotions and mind. There are aspects of living our lives that are akin to being in the best university imaginable, with the greatest professors, where we have the opportunity to learn about life and living, as well as self-acceptance, self-love, compassion, and healing. Do a great job in this area and when you encounter the stress, you will have healed and will have the "tools." At this point, the stress will no long trigger excessive emotional pain in you. And if it does trigger your own internal emotional pain, you'll be able to work with it in a safe and effective way.... on the spot, safely, quietly, and in the comfort and safety of your own emotions and mind. Also, once again and very important, the stress will not trigger the biology of the stress response in your body. Well, well, a huge and wonderful topic!

Thorough treatment of menopause often calls for the evaluation and treatment of hormones and organs beyond the ovaries. Systems that one would not think of as being related to menopause and health actually are. In medicine, "the knee bone is connected to the thigh bone, the thigh bone is connected to the hip bone... " Though menopause can primarily be thought of as an ovarian hormone event, proper treatment involves assessing and addressing other glands, hormones, neurotransmitters, liver, bones, nutrition, digestion, and more.

And alas, all systems of the body are not 20 years old anymore. We are dealing somewhere circa the "50,000-mile mark." The expected overall "wear and tear" is present and influential. Treating menopause goes beyond treating ovarian hormones.

 *"... the knee bone's connected to the thigh bone, the thigh bone's connected to the hip bone..."*

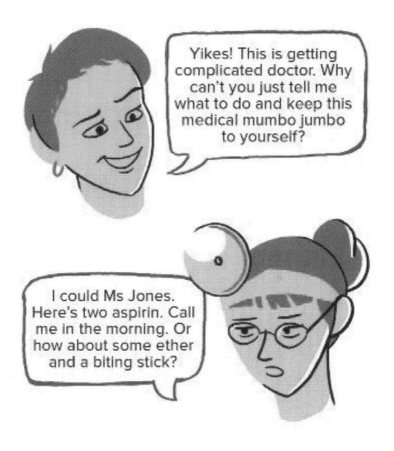

Chapter Five

# Initial Process and Evaluation

*Your Initial Evaluation is By You*

As always, it is best that you are the captain of your own health. You could be the first to know that something is amiss. The more sensitive and attuned you are to your own body, the sooner in perimenopause you will sense that something is changing. Regular cycles could become irregular. Occasional breast tenderness, fullness, or PMS could appear "out of the blue." Sleep, mood, energy, and/or libido could change. Warm or hot flashes could come on. In many patients, subtle or definitive symptoms will begin to appear that will make them go beyond suspecting to knowing that something is just not quite right. On the other hand, a certain percentage of women notice only that their menstrual periods have ceased. These women sometimes wonder, "What is the problem?" They do not necessarily sense one. As a physician, it is rare that I encounter these women for menopausal issues. I have heard many a story in working with older women for various reasons, and many of them have told me they never experienced any symptoms or noticed anything other than an absence of periods. Let it be known, however, that they too are vulnerable to the underlying diminishing of health from hormone insufficiency.

Working with so many women in menopause, I have also encountered many who have had plenty of symptoms, and they did not like it one bit! Even more significant from my perspective, are the deeper and detrimental changes that commonly occur in the bones, muscles, mind, vagina, bladder, arteries, and elsewhere—all related to hormonal declines. I encourage all women of menopausal age to look carefully into assessing and addressing some of the underlying issues that can occur from hormonal deficiency, whether they have symptoms or not. I assert it is crucial for some, very important for many, not so important for a few, and even contraindicated in rare instances. Treating women in menopause with bio-identical hormones can be a marvelous example of "an ounce of prevention is worth a ton of cure."

From another vantage point, it is quite common for women of perimenopausal or menopausal age not to encounter the classic symptoms of menopause, but they may have a variety of non-specific yet significant health issues. This can appear in many forms. The symptoms can include energy depletion, weight gain, sleep and mood disorders, hypertension, and even pain. These issues do not seem immediately related to menopause. One of the general principles I have found to be so valuable when working with women of menopausal age is to thoroughly address their hormones first, no matter how many health issues exist, and see how many of those original issues actually remain after treatment! Over and over again, I have been surprised by how much can be achieved with hormonal interventions. Many health conditions, even dramatic ones, have "melted away."

If somewhere along the way you conclude it is important that you be assessed and possibly receive hormone treatment, you will arrive at the need for a licensed health professional who can prescribe hormones. Because hormones are involved, prescriptions will become necessary. Perhaps of most importance, is the need to find a properly trained, trustworthy, and compassionate physician or nurse practitioner. If you have difficulty finding a qualified medical professional locally, you may need to travel a bit for the first in-person consultation. After that first visit, much of the hormone treatment process can be successfully managed by phone consultations, especially if you continue to see your personal primary care physician or gynecologist for the remainder of your female medical issues and annual exams. In many states, The Menopause Method has physicians and nurse practitioners who offer telemedicine. You can find additional information on page 47.

*Second Step: Finding a Physician or Nurse Practitioner*

As I mentioned earlier, knowledge and experience about treating women in menopause with bio-identical hormones are not yet universal or even widespread. Even though there are thousands of qualified physicians and nurse practitioners who are trained in and doing this work, relatively speaking, this is not a great number, and they may or may not be in your town! If you should need to have your appendix removed, a surgeon very qualified to do so will not be far from your neighborhood: this knowledge and training is widespread and has been for a long time. However, this is not the case at this stage of treatment of women in menopause.

You can be fortunate. It may be that your family physician, gynecologist, or nurse practitioner has excellent training and experience in this field. If so, you are "home free." If not, you will need to "go shopping" for a qualified practitioner.

So, where do you begin? There are a number of options to consider, including:

1. It is important to know what criteria to use when assessing a practitioner's qualifications. This is one of the purposes of this book. If you can learn which elements are important in the evaluation, treatment, and monitoring of menopause, you will be better able to evaluate if a health professional is going to be the right one to assist you.

2. Nowadays, as always, there are "good doctors." Some of their qualities are that they know what they know, they are humble and cognizant about what they don't know, and they are curious about assisting you, even if it requires "venturing into new territory." Our staff at The Menopause Method is here to assist physicians if they have an interest. We provide training programs and consultations for professionals. (Information is available at www.menopausemethod.com.)

3. Another option is to do some research and consider whether you are willing to travel for an initial in-person consultation, at least once. I assert that there is a well-trained and excellent menopause health professional not so far away from where you live. If you have difficulty finding a menopause and bio-identical hormone specialist, again, you can email us through "Find a Doc" at www.menopausemethod.com. We have trained many physicians and nurse practitioners in the United States. We will be happy to assist you with finding one in your area or within a reasonable distance, or, if possible, recommend one of our tele-medine-trained physicians or nurse practitioners.

4. You can contact your local compounding pharmacist and ask them who they recommend.

5. There are organizations that offer provider directories online. This can assist you in finding a practitioner in your area who specializes in bio-identical hormone treatment. If you have an interest, you could enter your zip code into the following websites: www.funtionalmedicine.org, www.A4M.com, and www.ACAM.org.

6. To learn more about a specific practitioner, you could contact their office. Most often, they will have a staff member designated to speak with potential new patients. Some practitioners will even speak with you themselves on the phone prior to scheduling a first appointment!

7. Telemedicine: Online live, HIPAA-secure, computer-based video consultations with a Menopause Method trained physician or nurse practitioner are now possible. Most often, an in-person office visit is not required. Ongoing blood and hormone testing can be carried out by requisition to local labs and hormone testing kits shipped to specialty labs. Important monitoring, including female exams, transvaginal ultrasounds, etc. can be performed by your local and favorite gynecologist or trained practitioner of female medicine. Breast imaging and bone evaluations can be done by your local radiologist. All examination and test results can be forwarded to your telemedicine hormone consultant professional. If you would like, our Menopause Method staff can often connect you with one of our trained practitioners licensed in your state. Please visit our website, www.menopausemethod.com/findadoc, for details.

If you need assistance from a medical professional, again, one of my intentions is that by the time you finish reading this book, you will have an understanding of what you should be looking for, and, just as important, what you do not want.

*The Next Step: Evaluation By Your Health Professional*

So much valuable information can be learned in an initial consultation by a practitioner of menopause medicine. A thorough medical history and physical exam can often bring to light many health concerns. Comprehensive medical questionnaires with an imbedded focus on female health are of special value. You can go to www.menopausemethod.com to view a sample of our questionnaire (this is for demonstration purposes only). There is a specific section that focuses on female health. One part of that section is structured in such a way that women can easily identify symptoms common to menopause (e.g., deficiencies of estrogen, progesterone, and testosterone). I am including that specific segment (Figure 5 on the next two pages) for your perusing and identifying pleasure. Perhaps you'll even "recognize" yourself.

*Other Initial Evaluations*

Basic blood tests are important, both routine testing and thyroid testing that includes TSH, free T3, free T4, and reverse T3. I also want to see the sex hormone binding globulin (SHBG) and vitamin D levels and, at times, DHEA-S along with free and total testosterone levels. Other blood tests are possible; the list can be long, depending on any additional health issues. Commonly, I will order a fasting insulin and hemoglobin A1C.

Figure 5. Initial Questionnaire: Assessment of Ovarian Hormones

### Symptoms of Estrogen Deficiency:

| Symptom | Value | | Symptom | Value |
|---|---|---|---|---|
| Hot flashes: | 2 | | Depression: | 3 |
| Warm rushes: | 2 | | Weight gain: | 3 |
| Night sweats: | 0 | | Trouble falling asleep: | 1 |
| Back and joint pain: | 5 | | Kicking covers off at night: | 5 |
| Vaginal dryness: | 5 | | Heart palpitations: | 5 |
| Mental fogginess: | 5 | | Chest pain: | 2 |
| Racing mind at night: | 1 | | Headaches and Migraines: | 2 |
| Intestinal bloating: | 3 | | Diminished sexuality and sensuality: | 4 |
| Hair loss: | 1 | | Pain on intercourse: | 3 |

### Symptoms of Estrogen Excess:

| Symptom | Value | | Symptom | Value |
|---|---|---|---|---|
| Breast tenderness: | 0 | | Water retention: | 1 |
| Nipple tenderness: | 2 | | Swelling: | 3 |
| Breast fullness: | 4 | | Impatient and snappy with clear mind: | 1 |
| Nausea: | 2 | | Breast swelling or enlargement: | 3 |
| Pelvic cramps: | 4 | | | |

### Symptoms of Progesterone Deficiency:

| Symptom | Value | | Symptom | Value |
|---|---|---|---|---|
| Difficulty sleeping: | 1 | | Anxiety and Nervousness: | 2 |
| Irregular period: | 3 | | Spotting before period: | 4 |
| Water retention: | 1 | | Infrequent period: | 3 |
| No period: | 4 | | Frequent and heavy periods: | 1 |
| Painful breasts: | 0 | | Fibrocystic breasts: | 1 |
| Fibroids: | 2 | | Endometriosis: | 3 |
| Diminished sex drive: | 4 | | PMS: | 1 |

Figure 5. Initial Questionnaire: Assessment of Ovarian Hormones, continued

Symptoms of Testosterone Deficiency:

| | | | |
|---|---|---|---|
| Diminished sex drive: | 0 | Diminished sense of security: | 0 |
| Indecisiveness: | 0 | Diminished aggressiveness: | 0 |
| Muscle weakness: | 0 | Diminished energy and stamina: | 0 |
| Muscle flabbiness: | 0 | Difficulty standing up from a squat: | 0 |
| Urine loss on cough: | 0 | Diminished coordination and balance: | 0 |
| Hair loss: | 0 | Diminished armpit, pubic, and/or body hair: | 0 |
| Diminished love of your body image: | 0 | | |

Baseline female exams, mammograms, bone density, and other assessments are often conducted if they haven't been performed on the patient recently. Other specific evaluations may be necessary as determined by the initial history and physical exam.

### What About Initial Hormone Testing?

Hormone testing is a topic I will address in significant detail in a later chapter. Interestingly, it is uncommon to need or find value in initial hormone testing in a perimenopausal or menopausal woman. After all, they are in the office because of symptoms of hormone depletion. In a menopausal woman, the best of the testing techniques will reveal little more than her hormone levels are *very low*, which has already been surmised from her history. During perimenopause, hormone levels can be very misleading because hormone output is often so erratic. With no ability to compare a woman's current hormone levels to her youthful levels, it cannot be determined how relatively low the levels are in comparison to her own "normal" at a younger age.

Thus, it is rare that I suggest initial ovarian hormone testing. I certainly did a lot of initial testing when I was first working with women in menopause. I quickly discovered that I did not learn anything of value. Invariably, hormone levels were very low. This was something I was already certain of based on their symptoms!

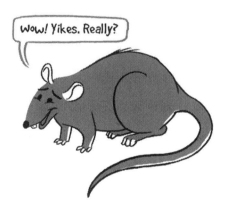

There are definitely exceptions. If a woman is curious and wants to know what her hormone levels are, and has no objection to the cost involved, that is fine. Also, if a woman seems to have unusual health issues, initial hormone testing may prove to be of value and unveil special depletions of androgens and/or corticosteroids that will need to be addressed early on.

Once a woman stabilizes on a treatment program, hormonal testing of the highest quality is crucial and imperative in my medical practice. To "name names," that would be the 24-hour urine hormone test. It is a test we always do, and we repeat it +/- annually thereafter.

Yet, the vast majority of the time, we suggest waiting until the woman and her practitioner agree that optimal hormone treatment has been achieved clinically. Important information will be learned from testing at that time.

Occasionally, we will test earlier in the process of dose discovery if programs are especially challenging and we need additional information along the way. We will go into the subject of hormonal testing in later chapters.

With the initial evaluations complete, we move on to discuss hormones and treatments.

Chapter Six

# Progesterone

### *Why Progesterone First?*

As I have mentioned, when a woman reaches her mid-30s or later, symptoms resulting from progesterone decline may be the first perimenopausal occurrence of significance. The word "progesterone" derives from "pro-gestational"—supportive of pregnancy. Progesterone levels skyrocket during pregnancy and are essential to sustain the pregnancy to full term. Adequate progesterone is also necessary to sustain the length of the menstrual cycle to 28 +/- days. Recall that in order to produce progesterone in any cycle, a woman must ovulate during that cycle. Should ovulation become erratic or even cease (thus, ovarian progesterone production cease), menstrual cycles can become irregular and often shorter. Deeper into perimenopause, the cycle length can become longer and even progress to the point of missing one or more periods.

The symptoms of estrogen dominance can emerge when adequate progesterone is not present to balance estrogen. As a result, the uterus and breasts can become overstimulated, and thus uterine cramps and breast tenderness can occur. Uterine fibroids and fibrocystic breast disease can even develop from excessive

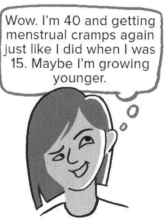

Wow. I'm 40 and getting menstrual cramps again just like I did when I was 15. Maybe I'm growing younger.

overstimulation of the uterus and breast glandular tissue.[6.1, 6.2] Of the 500,000 hysterectomies (surgical removal of the uterus) performed each year in the United States, primarily on 40 to 45-year-olds, 48% are because of uterine fibroids.[6.3] Fibroids, hysterectomies, and many oophorectomies (in this case, simultaneous removal of the ovaries) can often be prevented by identifying the decline of progesterone production and by restoring adequate progesterone[6.1] levels to rebalance the overstimulation by estrogen.

Progesterone also plays a significant role in maintaining healthy, strong bones, along with estrogens and other hormones and nutrients. Of importance is the fact that progesterone promotes bone health in a different way than estrogens: it stimulates osteoblasts, the cells that lay down new bone. With low progesterone levels, bones can lose the full advantage of stimulated new bone growth. As a result, osteopenia and/or osteoporosis can result.

As I emphasize time and again, it is remarkably practical for a woman and/or her health professional to be able to identify as early as possible a relative progesterone decline as well as the cessation of ovulation and treat with progesterone. By doing so, great good can be done!

*Recognize the decline*
*of progesterone,*
*restore it to reasonable levels,*
*and great good can be done!*

*Biochemistry of Progesterone*

Just for fun, I want to introduce you to "biochemical road maps." It's a language used by chemists, and it can be useful to you in understanding hormones. As you can see in Figure 6a, cholesterol is converted into the "great grand-mother" of steroid hormones, pregnenolone. Pregnenolone

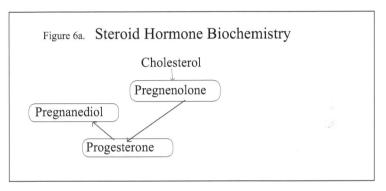

Figure 6a. Steroid Hormone Biochemistry

Cholesterol

Pregnenolone

Pregnanediol

Progesterone

in turn is converted into progesterone in both the ovaries and the adrenal glands. Ovarian progesterone then travels through the bloodstream and is taken up by many tissues: brain, bones, breasts, and others. It connects with the progesterone receptor sites in the cells of those tissues—and it has an effect on those cells. After the process of being utilized in the cell receptor sites, progesterone undergoes a biochemical conversion into a "metabolite" known as pregnanediol. Hormones, receptor sites, interaction, the process of utilization, and metabolization: we will see this pattern everywhere we look in the world of hormones. As part of our method to assess the amount of a hormone—in this case, progesterone—we often measure the amount of its metabolite(s). So, in this instance, we would measure its major metabolite, pregnanediol.

As I mentioned, in a young woman, the vast majority of progesterone is produced in the ovaries and in the cells that surround the egg that has been ovulated. Again, no ovulation, nil progesterone! In Figure 6b, I show an illustration of progesterone and estrogen as they appear during a menstrual cycle. This illustration would lead one to believe

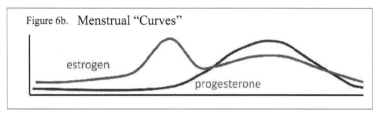

Figure 6b.  Menstrual "Curves"

estrogen

progesterone

that estrogen and progesterone were produced in relatively equal amounts. Not true. You will see in the more accurate graph (Figure 6c) that during the mid-luteal phase of a cycle (day 21 of a 28-day cycle, which is halfway between ovulation and menstruation) estrogen production in an ova-

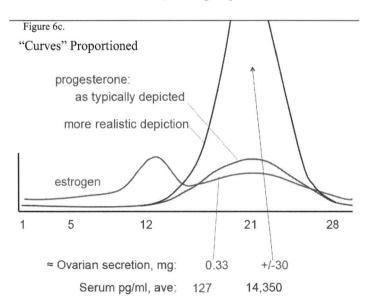

Figure 6c.

"Curves" Proportioned

progesterone:
    as typically depicted

more realistic depiction

estrogen

| | 1 | 5 | 12 | 21 | 28 |

≈ Ovarian secretion, mg:  0.33    +/-30

Serum pg/ml, ave:  127    14,350

ry is approximately 0.3 milligrams per day. In contrast, progesterone production is approximately +/- 30 milligrams per day. I mention this just so you can have a perspective of the value the body places on progesterone! Progesterone has received less recognition than is appropriate for the heroine that it is.

Once again, 50 years ago, it was believed that as a woman approached menopausal age, ovulation and menstruation ceased at the same time. Nowadays, that still occurs in some women. However, it is very common for ovulation to cease prior to the cessation of menstruation, even up to 10 years prior. I cannot emphasize enough that if you can identify an early progesterone decline from the emergence of progesterone deficiency symptoms (e.g., sleep and mood challenges, irregular periods, PMS, breast tenderness, etc.) and receive treatment with progesterone, it can be so beneficial for you. Substantial estrogen decline will eventually occur. Periods will cease, and it may be the time to supplement with estrogen. That time will occur in your far or near future.

## Progesterone Treatment

Biochemically identical molecules to ovarian progesterone have long been available. Interestingly enough, the plant world has many similarities to us humans. One such similarity is that many plants contain steroid hormones that are identical to our own. Or, shall we say, ours are identical to theirs. Some plants are richer in these hormones than others: soy and yam have the richest amount of relatively easily extractable steroids in the plant kingdom.

The pharmaceutical world was the first to popularize the production of an altered type of progesterone. This industry shied away from the natural form of progesterone because law prohibits the patenting of any molecule that is present in the human body. Without the exclusivity of patents, huge profits are not possible. Thus, the "progestins" were developed. They are significantly different from bio-identical progesterone molecularly and in how they behave physiologically. Progestins are at the foundation of most birth control pills and were the component in Prempro (the Premarin-progestins combination developed to treat women in menopause) that was found to be related to the increased incidence of serious diseases as revealed by the WHI scientific study. On the other hand, the medical literature shows us that bio-identical progesterone provides protection!

Bio-identical progesterone has been available for decades. In the mid-1990s, John Lee, M.D., was the first to extol the virtues and the crucial importance of natural progesterone. Through his work, there was widespread distribution of natural progesterone, at least through the health-conscious world. For decades, there has been 1.8% (mild) progesterone cream available over-the-counter, often found in "health food" stores. It has done so much good and can continue to do so, certainly when called for at the time of perimenopause. However, I do find this cream is generally not strong enough to produce the levels of progesterone that I would consider to be optimal as women move deeper into menopause. Often, over time, and if the skin loses its ability to absorb hormones, we will need to move on to stronger formulations. My favorite progesterone to begin with is suspended in an organic oils-based mixture, 200 mg/ml = 9 mg/drop. Gels and creams are also available, beginning at 3% and going up as high as 20%. In some instances, primarily due to absorption issues, we will change to an oral "micronized" form of dosing or, for some, a translabial or transperianal mucosa application. Sublingual applications can also be used.

Part of the reason for the absorption challenge is that the ovary, as we touched upon earlier, produced approximately +/- 30 milligrams of progesterone in its heyday, compared to 0.3–0.5 milligrams of estrogen. It is helpful for you to understand that though it can be relatively easy to absorb 0.5 milligrams of estrogen, +/- 30 milligrams of progesterone could present a greater challenge, simply because of the higher number of milligrams in progesterone — 60 times as much.

When treating with estrogen or testosterone, oral administration is shunned for significant important reasons. This is not so for progesterone. Sometimes we take advantage of a unique biochemistry that occurs in the metabolic processing of oral progesterone, which has special benefit in remedying sleep disturbance.

To summarize, below are my favorite forms of progesterone:

- 200 mg/ml progesterone in an organic oils-base
- 1.8% cream that is available "over the counter"
- 3% or 10% progesterone in a carbopol gel
- 20% progesterone cream in a lipoderm base
- 25, 50, 75, and 100 mg oral micronized progesterone

I will describe how to discover your optimal progesterone dose as well as administration methods further on in this book.

All of the above formulations are prepared by "compounding pharmacies." Compounding pharmacies are the "old-fashioned" type. They carry the traditional patent medicines, as do all pharmacies. In addition, their pharmacists formulate custom made-to-order prescriptions as specified by physicians and other practitioners who are licensed to prescribe. They have likely been in your neighborhood for years; you may or may not have known about them. They definitely were the first to become interested in bio-identical hormones and have often been doing this work for three to four decades. I have benefited from their interest, dedication, knowledge, experience, and expertise.

To date, there are no commercial transdermal progesterone products available other than the over-the-counter, lower-dose creams that I have mentioned earlier. There is an oral form, called Prometrium®, that is prepared by a pharmaceutical manufacturer. It contains micronized progesterone, peanut oil, and a few chemicals in a capsule and is available only in 100 and 200 milligram dosages. Because of these large dosages, the use of peanut oil, and the chemical additives, I have never prescribed it.

# Chapter Seven

# Estrogens

*A Family of Hormones: Rx, Bi-Est*

I have introduced you to the qualities of estrogen and the symptoms of estrogen deficiency. "Estrogen" is the name given to a *family of hormones* and is *not* the name of a specific hormone. However, this word is often used inter-changeably as if it were a specific hormone. Below are the three most clinically active forms of the estrogens:

- Estradiol (E2): This is the principle estrogen hormone produced and secreted by the ovary. It is the most potent in this family of hormones.

- Estrone (E1): This is a common form of estrogen, and it is about 80% as potent and twice as prevalent as E2. It is the main form that is transported in the blood stream.

- Estriol (E3): This is a hormonally active metabolite of E1, and it is about 1/8th as potent as E2.

Let's look at an estrogen biochemical "roadmap" that follows:

Estradiol (E2) ⇌ Estrone (E1)

Estriol (E3)

## Historical Note

When the treatment of women in menopause with estrogen-active substances began in earnest in the United States (in the 1940s), the commercial pharmaceutical product Premarin® was being marketed. Interestingly, Premarin consists of "conjugated equine estrogens" (CEEs) that are derived from the urine of pregnant mares. Of significance is the fact that 50% of the hormones found in Premarin are different than those found in human females, and they are foreign to the female body. This was the beginning of mass production and widespread use of estrogens. Looking back, it is understandable why they chose what seems to be an unlikely source of estrogen compounds: they were able to procure large quantities of the horse urine and then extract the estrogens from it.

Many years ago, I was having lunch with a compounding pharmacist. He asked me if I had ever wondered why the covering on a Premarin pill was so thick. He told me that he once was curious, bit into it, and quickly encountered a heavy odor of urine! Premarin became the number one income grossing pharmaceutical product and remained so for years. I could say more about equine estrogens but will choose to "hold my tongue." CEE's sales dropped dramatically after the WHI publication revealed increased risks. Recall that the increased risks were not associated with Premarin use alone but only with the use of Premarin in combination with a progestin, Provera®. In recent years, pharmaceutical companies have been producing estradiol-based estrogen products.

Decades before the WHI, a pioneer physician, Jonathan Wright, MD, came up with the novel idea of using "exact molecular copies" of human estrogens, as he knew these estrogens were being extracted from plants and were available in a pure form. Thus, began the use of "bio-identical" hormones in the early 1980s.

Dr. Wright also pointed out that "Nature" had specific ratios of E1, E2, and E3 in young women and that we should prescribe in a way to copy that pattern. He cited a 24-hour urine hormone study done on both healthy women and women who had breast cancer, noting that the women who had breast cancer had significantly less estriol (E3) in their urine than healthy women.[7.1]

Many physicians learning from Dr. Wright and others, myself included, have stayed with this estrogen formulation. Interestingly enough, research in the last five years has added very strong evidence to the importance of estriol. Details have emerged on the proliferation-stimulating estrogen receptor alpha (ERα) and the anti-proliferative estrogen receptor beta (ERβ), along with the special affinity estriol has for ERβ.[7.2] The cells in breast glandular tissue have both of these receptor sites. As a menstrual cycle progresses towards ovulation, the proliferative effects of ERα predominate and cells are added in preparation for possible breast milk production. If fertilization does not occur, the ERβ effects of de-proliferation (cell demise through "apoptosis") predominate, and the breast fullness that was developing recedes.

What's more, though estradiol interacts with both ERα and ERβ, estriol has a significant preference for interaction with ERβ. Thus, estriol is a discourager of breast glandular proliferation: exactly what we want in treating women in menopause!

$$\boxed{\text{Bi-Est} = \text{E3} + \text{E2}}$$

Therefore, my preferred estrogen formulation is "Bi-Est." It is a combination of estriol and estradiol. Our ultimate goal is to prescribe the proper Bi-Est formulation that will result in urine levels of E1, E2, and E3 that "copy Nature." Dr. Wright has shown us that the following fraction ("estrogen quotient" [EQ]) is generated from the micrograms of each hormone excreted in the urine in 24 hours:

$$\boxed{EQ = \frac{E3}{E2 + E1} \geq 2}$$

Thus, this formulation contains estriol in at least twice the quantity of the sum of estradiol + estrone. This ratio is challenged by some,[7.3] stating that in young women this ratio is closer to "1" than to "2." Regardless, this still calls for a rich amount of estriol in any formulation. The studies citing the importance of E3 with respect to ERβ keep me a proponent of rich levels of estriol, but not too much, in any given Bi-Est prescription. My optimal EQ is between 2 and 4... taking into account other details in the 24-hour urine hormone test, as well as a woman's sense of well-being.

Most often this is achieved from an original prescription that includes 80% E3 + 20% E2. I prescribe this formulation for all of my initial Bi-Est Rx's. Occasionally, after reviewing the symptoms of a newly treated patient, or after viewing the results of the 24-hour urine hormone test and finding an EQ that is higher than 4, I'll change the percentages in my Rx to 70:30, 60:40, or 50:50. This will increase the amount of E2 and decrease the amount of E3, thus decrease the EQ... and often improve my patient's symptoms. At other times, if the EQ is > 4, but the patient is very content and the estrogen metabolites are fine, I will not change the formulation. This will result in a more robust E3 than usual. That can be desirable considering the benefit for the ERβ (estrogen receptor site beta) and its emphasis on de-proliferation. If this seems staggeringly complex to you, no worries: this level of detail is in the province of your medical professional.

So, why is there no estrone (E1) in the Bi-Est formulation? Testing reveals that if you prescribe E2 and E3, sufficient E1 will appear in the urine hormone test results. Because of the manner in which biochemical processing takes place, it is not necessary to prescribe E1... Nature's proportions will develop internally.

There is more to prescribing Bi-Est, and it depends on the strength of the formulation. The stronger (more concentrated) the formulation, the less oil, cream, or gel is needed to apply to the skin, vagina, or external perianal mucosa with each hormone application. Also, the stronger the formulation, the less the monthly expense will be for the patient! This is because the cost involved in compounding hormones is mostly related to the labor required. Thus, it is no more expensive to make a formulation two times any strength.

Let me give you an example of this. Again, the most common formulation of Bi-Est I prescribe is 30 mg/ml 80:20 (80% E3, 20% E2). Let's say that after a few months of dose discovery, a woman is applying 4 drops twice a day and is very content with the symptom relief. By doubling the strength of her next prescription to Bi-Est 60 mg/ml 80:20, she can replicate her optimal dose by applying 2 drops twice a day. This new Rx, for the *same* price as the previous Rx, lasts her twice as long!

This dose alteration does have limitations, however. Let's say a woman was content with 2 drops twice daily of Bi-Est 30 mg/ml. I would *not* then prescribe 1 drop twice daily of Bi-Est 60 mg/ml. I would stay with the original 30 mg/ml formulation. Here are the reasons why:

- 2 or 3 drops is the ideal amount of drops to apply to the skin with each dosage. The utter optimal amount of Bi-Est is 2 drops in the a.m. and 3 drops in the p.m. or vice versa: "3 & 2."
  - o 4 or more drops is a bit much of an amount of Bi-Est in oils to apply to the skin at any one time.
  - o 1 drop is not okay: again, should a woman need to add an extra drop for any reason, such as increased estrogen need at a time of stress, 1 additional drop represents too great an increment in total dosage to be working with at a given time of dose increase.

To summarize, considering the strength of a formulation and cost per month to the patient for any given hormone Rx:

- The optimal amount of Bi-Est or testosterone in oils to apply to the skin at any one given time is 2 or 3 drops.
- Once the optimal dosage is discovered through titration, physicians and nurse practitioners will often adjust the strength of Bi-Est to have the final outcome

translate into 2 or 3 drops per application. They also take into account that it is desirable to increment the dosage of a single drop by a small amount should you desire to add an extra drop.

- This principle of optimizing formula strength and the number of drops will also apply to choosing the formulation for transperianal or vaginal application of an oils formulation. This time, however, fewer drops are more optimal to apply to these mucosal surfaces.

- When using a total of 5 drops of Bi-Est daily, the bottle will last one month! Fancy math: there are 162 drops per Rx bottle. 2 drops in the a.m. plus 3 drops in the p.m. = 5 drops per day. Thus, 162 drops per bottle ÷ 5 drops per day = 32 days' worth of Rx per bottle. You will be stopping the Bi-Est application once a month for 2, 3, or 4 days, so you will have a one-month supply.

- Pharmacists are accustomed to pricing prescriptions on a per-month basis.

- After you determine your initial dose, a Menopause Method trained physician will calculate the Bi-Est strength to optimize mg/ml and deliver 5 drops per day: 2 in the a.m. and 3 in the p.m., or 3 in the a.m. and 2 in the p.m. Other adjustments to the estriol and estradiol ratio may be made upon receiving the results of the 24-hour urine hormone test. This fine-tuning optimizes health experience and safety.

- Transdermal progesterone in oils is handled differently. 95% of all progesterone in oils prescriptions are 200 mg/ml, which is the concentration maximum per ml. This robust strength is required because a woman's body has such a need for more progesterone, milligram-for-milligram, as compared to Bi-Est or testosterone. When a woman is using transdermal progesterone, it is not unusual for her to titrate up to 6 drops per night. Yes, this can be a lot of oil, which also happen to have benefit to the skin, by design. For a woman who has skin that is very absorbent, transdermal progesterone works well.We can measure this absorption in the 24-hour urine hormone test. As a woman's skin ages and potentially becomes less absorbent over time (which is observable in the hormone test results), we will change to an oral dosage form of progesterone. If a woman has special need for sleep improvement that is not accomplished by the initial replenishment of ovarian hormones, we will often prescribe oral progesterone as it can have special additional sleep benefit.

• These same principles can be applied to gels and creams as we go to balance the strength and ratio of the formulation with symptoms and the hormone test results.

You will reply on your knowledgeable health professional to sort out, prescribe, and account for these details.

*There is an important guideline to follow regarding estrogen dosing: whatever the total daily dose you are prescribed and titrate to, we always suggest that you divide that dose into two daily applications. It is important that you do not try to consolidate that dose into one application per day, so as to avoid one single, abrupt rise in blood estrogen (known as "peaking"). For this reason, we divide estrogen into two smaller rises per day.*

Here are my favorite transdermal preparations to start with as the initial prescription:

- Bi-Est: 30 mg/ml 80:20 in the proprietary organic oils-blend formulation and delivery system. By far, this is my number one preference! Any compounding pharmacist who wants to dispense with this base can obtain it from www.menopausemethod.com by selecting "For Pharmacists."

- Bi-Est: 2.5 mg/ml 80:20 or 2.75 mg/ml 73:27 in a carbopol or other solvent base preferred by your compounding pharmacy.

In addition, I recommend that estrogens should *not* be given orally for a number of reasons, which include:

- Potential increase in blood coagulability and inflammation[7.4]

- Production of excessive metabolites in the "first pass through the liver"[7.5] effect

*The increase in blood coagulability and inflammation are the most significant possible consequences of oral administration of estrogens. For example, the main problem with arteriosclerosis is the possibility of a clot forming on the irregular atherosclerotic surface of an artery, which can be fatal.7.6 Thus, we value anything that does not potentially increase coagulability. Also to be considered is that when a hormone like estradiol (or Premarin) is swallowed, it is absorbed, and then circulated directly to the liver. In the liver, a high percentage of the hormone is converted into metabolites, while only a percentage of it flows through the liver as untouched estradiol. This is the so-called "first pass through the liver effect." Next, the estradiol and metabolites leave the liver and circulate onward to the remainder of the body. This is quite different from how the ovary functions: estradiol is secreted directly into the bloodstream, goes onward to the entire body and, then, it is finally picked up by the liver and metabolized. Applying hormones to the skin mimics the ovary in that the hormones are taken up directly by the blood and circulated to the body, and then are metabolized.*

*Another upshot of the oral administration of estradiol is that an excessive dosage is required for a sufficient portion of estrogen to leave the liver unmetabolized. In this process, excessive metabolites are produced.*

Let's move on to learn how to find your optimal dosages!

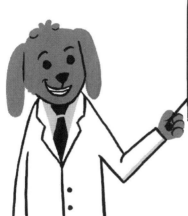

Before we go further into the treatment of menopause, there is even more background information that will bevaluable to consider. As mentioned earlier, menopause beigns, or derzarcated when ovarian horomone production of endrogen, progestrone, and testosterne falls below a certin threshold. When ovulation ceases, progestertan production will fallto very low levels in all women. However, individual women produce differing amounts ofestrogen. In some women estrogen can diminish gradually, "slipping" belowan adiquate enough to produce a significant uterine lineing (and there will be no possibility of mensturation). Their estrogen in this one, may still be presentin unobstructed though lesser amounts. Women who experiance this gradual decline seem to have an easier tyme with fewer symptoms... During menopause birth control pill is another serious factor that contributes to accessive estrogen stimulation. "The pill" contains certin horomones that have a different molecular structure than nautual horomones. Because of the artifical pact of the molecules htye will require additional lver processingbirth control pills contain only aggressive

# Chapter Eight

# Hormone Dose Determination

*You're Evaluated and Ready to Begin*

By the end of your first appointment with your physician or nurse practitioner, you will likely be receiving a prescription and instructions for your next phase. I mention "phase" because replenishing hormones and addressing other aspects of menopause is a process. As I illustrated in Chapter Two (Figure 2a), hormone levels decline as a woman ages. Hormonal decline is a process in itself that takes place over decades. Because every significant biological change in your body is accompanied by many internal adjustments and compensations from the time hormonal decline began in your twenties until now, many internal re-arrangements have taken place during your lifetime. Any strategy of restoration should have both short and long-term readjustments. It is a process that has different phases; it takes place over time and should not be hurried. As you begin treatment with hormones, your body will be making a new series of adjustments. So, lean back, take your time, and enjoy... good things are most likely "a comin!"

"Hormone dose determination": what the heck is that?! I gave you a preview of this earlier when I spoke of "shadowing" Dr. Gaby and learning about one of his patients who was going to begin finding her own dose of thyroid hormone. This is what you will be doing with ovarian hormones in an optimal treatment program. The difference is that you will be discovering optimal dosages beginning with first two hormones and, eventually, an additional two over time.

I'd like to illustrate. Below is an example of a typical patient reporting back to her doctor after being taught how to find her optimal dose of thyroid hormone:

"Well Doctor, I took one thyroid hormone pill each morning for the first 10 days like you told me, and I didn't notice a thing. The second 10 days, I increased my dose to 1.5 pills each morning, and... gosh, I wasn't sure. Beginning with the third 10 days, I started taking 2 pills a day. I did notice quite a change, and I liked it. During the fourth 10 days, I increased my dose once more to 2.5 pills every morning, and after a few days, I noticed that I was even feeling better on 2.5 pills than I was feeling on 2. Eventually, I increased my dose to 3 pills a day, and within three days, I became nervous, jittery, had heart palpitations, couldn't sleep, and developed a tremor. Just like you warned me, these were obviously symptoms of an excessive dose. So, I cut down to 2.5 pills a day and soon felt fine. After a while, just for curiosity, I wanted to see how I would feel on 2 pills a day. I felt okay on 2 pills but soon returned to 2.5 pills a day. My correct dose is 2.5 pills per day, Doctor!"

Here, we have the classic example of a patient finding her own dose from the feel of what was going on in her own body through a process known as "titration." Our next step in evaluating her thyroid hormone status would be to test her thyroid blood levels to confirm the levels are within optimal range.

Titration is a process of starting with a lowish dose and gradually increasing the amount of the dose until symptoms of hormonal insufficiency are alleviated. During this process, we are careful to stay shy of symptoms of hormonal excess or to back down the dosage if symptoms of excess occur. The difference in menopause is that you have more than one hormone to determine. No worries. Thousands of women have found their way through this process. Your health professional will give you a specific and clear road map. Eventually, your hormones will be tested to confirm you have arrived at optimal dosages.

> *Titration is a process*
> *of starting with a lowish dose*
> *and gradually increasing the amount*
> *of the dose until the symptoms*
> *of hormonal insufficiency are alleviated.*
> *All the while, we are careful*
> *to stay shy of symptoms*
> *of hormonal excess or*
> *to back down the dosage*
> *if symptoms of excess are reached.*

To be successful at titration, a prime requisite is that you have a familiarity with the symptoms of insufficiency and excess (see Figure 8a on the next page). Most women are beginning this process with one, two, or more clear-cut symptoms of insufficiency; that is why they are embarking on a program. There are exceptions when symptoms are more vague. Dose determination by titration then becomes a bit more subtle. More often than not, there is something that is mightily clear, such as several hot flashes during the day and also during the night!

---

### Deficiency Symptoms of Progesterone and Estrogen

**PROGESTERONE**                                      Figure 8a.

**Too little:**

- Sleep disturbance*
- Increased anxiety
- Mood disturbances
  (sometimes severe)
- Hot flashes*
- Breast tenderness*
- New &/or enlarged breast lumps

- Water retention*
- Difficulty relaxing
- Decreased libido*
- Period irregularities
  (if still menstruating)
- PMS, fibroids, &/or
  endometriosis

---

**ESTROGENS**

Too little:

- Warm rushes
- Night sweats
- Sleep disturbance*
- Mental fogginess
  &/or forgetfulness
- Weight gain (primarily
  thighs, hips &/or buttocks)
- Dry vagina, eyes &/or skin
- Diminished sensuality
  & sexuality*
- Sense of normalcy only
  during 2nd week (if cycling)

- Hot flashes*
- Temperature swings
- Racing mind at night
- Fatigue or reduced stamina
- Episodes of rapid heartbeat
  &/or palpitations
- Pain during intercourse
- Loss of glow
- Back &/or joint pain
- Intestinal bloating
- Headaches &/or migraines

---

Your physician or nurse practitioner will often initiate the treatment process by giving you:

- a customized prescription for Bi-Est and/or progesterone;

- instructions regarding your starting dosage;

- information on *how much* to increase each dose; and

- information on *when* to increase each dose.

To know the upper limit of dosages, you will need to be familiar with the symptoms of excess for that specific hormone. I will repeat the symptoms of insufficiency for estrogens and progesterone as well as the symptoms of excess in the charts that follow.

*Perimenopausal Progesterone*

I am writing this book today because of an experience I had 23 years ago. One of my patients, Debra, arrived for a consultation and changed an aspect of the course of my career. She exclaimed that she was terribly upset and angrily said to me, "Don't pretend you think you know me and that I really am alright. I'm not, and this is major. I feel like I'm going crazy."

At that time, I had serendipitously had conversations with a pioneer in menopausal medicine, John Lee, MD, as well as a nearby compounding pharmacist that I continue to work with to this day. Dr. Lee emphasized the importance of progesterone. And, as it turned out, Tom White, RPh, told me he had transdermal progesterone. After initiating progesterone treatment with Debra, she called me three weeks later a "different person." She exclaimed, "Thank you. I'm back!" That was impressive to me as well: so much good had been done by so little effort! My medical practice was at the beginning of taking a whole new direction.

And, so many women, like Debra, have treasured the benefits of improved sleep and mood from progesterone.

If you are early in perimenopause, progesterone may be the only hormone you are likely to be prescribed. Perhaps you are experiencing a progesterone deficiency symptom such as sleep dysfunction that is new to you. Or, maybe you are moodier than you have ever been in your entire life. Maybe you are experiencing breast tenderness or irregular periods. Until you develop symptoms of estrogen deficiency as well, it would be common to begin treatment with progesterone alone. I have emphasized many times the value of identifying the relative earlier and more significant decline of progesterone than estrogen—as early as possible—and treating with progesterone.

For example, I would recommend that an early perimenopausal woman begins by rubbing 3 drops of progesterone 200 mg/ml (= 26 mg) into her skin at bedtime. I also recommend that she continues to increase it by 1 drop every three to five nights until she touches upon symptoms of excess and then back down the dose. Hopefully, along the way, she will feel the benefits, such as improved sleep and mood. If she then desires additional daytime mood improvement, I'd suggest adding a drop or two or more in the morning as well. This starting dose and rate of adding an additional drop—every three to five days—is a more aggressive plan than I suggest for a woman in menopause, as you will soon see. A total of 6 drops is a substantial amount of oil to apply at any one time. If progesterone insufficiency symptoms are not alleviated or 24-hour urine hormone test results ultimately do not show adequate progesterone absorption, we then often utilize another form of progesterone such as oral capsules. I will describe these further on.

It is most common to take the entire dose of progesterone at bedtime. We are not concerned about the spiking of progesterone as we are with estrogen. As I mentioned, a daytime dose of progesterone could benefit mood, yet some women will become drowsy from taking any progesterone during the day. These are the kind of determinations a woman will make by feeling the differences, or not.

In Figure 8b below, you will find a more extensive chart showing the symptoms of progesterone insufficiency and excess. Here, you will find the parameters of "too little" and "too much" as you discover your optimal dose.

---

Figure 8b.

**Finding Your Optimal Dose**

**PROGESTERONE**

Too little:
- Sleep disturbance*
- Increased anxiety
- Mood disturbances
  (sometimes severe)
- Hot flashes*
- Breast tenderness*
- New &/or enlarged breast lumps
- Water retention*
- Difficulty relaxing
- Decreased libido*
- Period irregularities
  (if still menstruating)
- PMS, fibroids, &/or
  endometriosis

Too much:
- Drowsiness
- Waking up groggy &/or edgy
- Sense of physical instability
- Hot flashes* (if very excessive dose!)
- Feeling depressed
- Slight dizziness
- Leg discomfort/pain
- Water retention*

The Menopause Method

---

*Menopausal Bi-Est*

In the scenario I am about to describe, I'll be starting treatment with Bi-Est for a menopausal woman who is experiencing hot flashes. Here, is a common way that treatment begins: in many cases the patient's symptoms of progesterone deficiency were of gradual onset and were not uncomfortable enough to inspire her to seek assistance. But, eventually, hot flashes may appear, awaken her in the night, disturb sleep, and are disruptive enough that her interest is fully kindled. Research is done, a health professional is found, and an appointment is made. Most commonly, we begin treatment with Bi-Est and progesterone at the same time: most women do just fine with beginning both hormones at once. Occasionally, we begin with Bi-Est alone as this provides an opportunity to get an "internal feel" for what Bi-Est feels like by itself before adding progesterone.

One of our prime objectives, if at all possible, is to have you get an internal feel for each hormone. By doing so, you

---

**Finding Your Optimal Dose**                                    Figure 8c.

**ESTROGENS**

**Too little:**
- Warm rushes
- Night sweats
- Sleep disturbance*
- Mental fogginess
  &/or forgetfulness
- Weight gain (primarily
  thighs, hips &/or buttocks)
- Dry vagina, eyes &/or skin
- Diminished sensuality
  & sexuality*
- Sense of normalcy only
  during 2nd week (if cycling)

- Hot flashes*
- Temperature swings
- Racing mind at night
- Fatigue or reduced stamina
- Episodes of rapid heartbeat
  &/or palpitations
- Pain during intercourse
- Loss of glow
- Back &/or joint pain
- Intestinal bloating
- Headaches &/or migraines

**Too much:**
- Breast tenderness*
- Breast fullness
- Impatient but clear of mind
- Pelvic cramps (w or
  w/o bleeding)

- Nipple tenderness
- Malaise
- Water retention (swollen
  fingers, legs &/or ankles)
- Hot flashes* (if excessive dose!)

---

*\* These symptoms can have more than one cause.*
*When in doubt, call your doctor*

**Do not exceed your doctor's suggested maximum dosages**

 the**menopause**method    For important instructions on how to apply hormones, go to:
*www.menopausemethod.com/application*

---

will be able to make minor adjustments to your protocol simply "by feel" if need be. Someday in the future, you may proclaim, "Ah, I feel like I might be a tad low on estrogen. I think I'll adjust my dose upward a smidgen." One of the main ways you can get a feel for where you stand regarding dosage is to learn the symptoms of insufficiency and excess. In The Menopause Method, your physician or nurse practitioner will give you a card (as pictured on the two preceding pages) that specifies these symptoms.

So, let's use an example of a 52-year-old, 5'5", 125 lb. woman who has not had a period for six months. She has an average of five hot flashes during the day along with three that awaken her at night. Let's say she has never experienced any particular sensitivity to medications that would require her to take "a quarter of what anyone else would take." Typically, I would start her on the following regimen:

- Bi-Est 30 mg/ml (80% E3: 20% E2) in the proprietary organic oils base
  o 1 drop in the morning and
  o 1 drop at bedtime
  o Rubbed into the soft part of her forearms

**Most Common Starting Rx**

patient _____ date _____

Bi-Est 30 mg/ml 80:20  8.5 ml  gtts 1–3 b.i.d.
Progesterone 200 mg/ml  8.5 ml  gtts 2–6 h.s.

B·E = Bi-Est | P = Progesterone

Number of Drops:

| | a.m. | p.m. | |
|---|---|---|---|
| days | B·E | B·E | P |
| 1 to 7 | 1 | 1 | 2 |
| 8 to 14 | 1 | 2 | 3 |
| 15 to 21 | 2 | 2 | 4 |
| 22 to 28 | 2 | 3 | 5 |
| 29 to – | 3 | 3 | 6 |

In The Menopause Method, physicians and nurse practitioners also give their patients *one* of four initial dose cards that relate to their specific protocol. Above is an example of the "Most Common Starting Rx" for our 52-year-old woman.

I'd suggest that she stay on that dose of "1 and 1 drops" for seven days and that she does not try to consolidate the dose into 2 drops once per day... as this seems to be a common inclination. As you may recall, we always want to divide estrogen dosages into twice daily applications so as to avoid one single abrupt rise ("spike") in estrogen levels, which occurs with once daily application.

Let's say that by the end of the first seven days of treatment her hot flashes have reduced to two in the daytime and one or two at night. Though her symptoms have improved, they have not been sufficiently alleviated. So, next, we would recommend that she increase her nighttime dose to 2 drops while keeping her morning dose at 1 drop. We prefer to first increase the nighttime dose, as alleviating middle-of-the-night, sleep-disturbing hot flashes is our higher priority. Note that I am suggesting the Bi-Est dosage can be increased every seven days — and to avoid the temptation to increase it more rapidly. There can be exceptions,

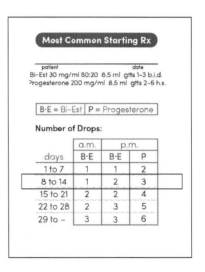

**Most Common Starting Rx**

patient        date
Bi-Est 30 mg/ml 80:20  8.5 ml  gtts 1-3 b.i.d.
Progesterone 200 mg/ml  8.5 ml  gtts 2-6 h.s.

B·E = Bi-Est | P = Progesterone

Number of Drops:

| | a.m. | p.m. | |
|---|---|---|---|
| days | B·E | B·E | P |
| 1 to 7 | 1 | 1 | 2 |
| 8 to 14 | 1 | 2 | 3 |
| 15 to 21 | 2 | 2 | 4 |
| 22 to 28 | 2 | 3 | 5 |
| 29 to – | 3 | 3 | 6 |

but that should be left to the guidance of your physician, nurse practitioner, or prescribing compounding pharmacist.

After a week on this new regimen, with an increase of 1 drop of Bi-Est in the evening (1 and 2 drops per day), let's say that she no longer experienced any hot flashes, day or night. Let's also say that she had not developed any breast or nipple tenderness or excessive breast fullness, as these are symptoms of an excessive dose. Bravo! This is a simple example of how things can work. It's not always this easy and rapid, yet this can occur. I promise to give you some more challenging examples as we go on.

There is a fine point in using the oil. This oils blend is 100% organic and contains no solvents. Ovarian hormones are poorly soluble, even in an oils base. Thus, this blend is a suspension rather than a solution. For this reason, it requires a very thorough shaking of the bottle (5 to 8 vigorous shakes). At that point, you open the cap, tilt the bottle totally upside down over your forearm, and wait for that first drop. It often takes a moment for that first drop to emerge. If you are using more than 1 drop, the 2nd, 3rd, etc. will follow the first one quite quickly. For a video demonstration on hormone application and titration, see our website, www.menopausemethod.com.

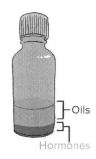

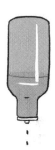

Again, there are other forms of transdermal hormones: gels and creams. I always begin with the organic oils as they are my favorite and contain no solvents or other chemicals. Ninety-five percent of my patients do well with the oils and never change to another formulation.

*Menopausal Progesterone*

With respect to timing again, there are two ways to treat with progesterone. One is to initiate progesterone treatment at the same time we begin Bi-Est. The other is to wait five to ten days, more or less, to see if a woman can discern what estrogen feels like on its own. However, because progesterone is always going to be used in the treatment of a menopausal woman, most often, we will start both hormones at the same time.

We begin by giving progesterone at night only. Typically, I would start a menopausal woman on the following program:

- Progesterone 200 mg/ml in the organic oils proprietary blend

  o 2 drops at bedtime, taken with nighttime Bi-Est

  o Apply to a different location on the body, such as the inner thighs (do not apply progesterone to the same areas as estrogen)

  o No progesterone in the morning

**Most Common Starting Rx**

patient _____ date _____
Bi-Est 30 mg/ml 80:20  8.5 ml  gtts 1-3 b.i.d.
Progesterone 200 mg/ml  8.5 ml  gtts 2-6 h.s.

B·E = Bi-Est | P = Progesterone

Number of Drops:

| days | a.m. | p.m. | |
|---|---|---|---|
| | B·E | B·E | P |
| 1 to 7 | 1 | 1 | 2 |
| 8 to 14 | 1 | 2 | 3 |
| 15 to 21 | 2 | 2 | 4 |
| 22 to 28 | 2 | 3 | 5 |
| 29 to – | 3 | 3 | 6 |

I'd suggest that she remain on that dose for one week. If she did not awaken in the morning with a symptom of progesterone overdose (see the previous chart, Figure 8b, page 79), she would then increase the dose to 3 drops at bedtime on days 8 to 14.

Over time, a woman can keep increasing her progesterone dose as necessary. Ultimately, she will eventually be able to make adjustments to her progesterone dose independently of her estrogen dosing. In the previous example, we have a scenario where hot flashes have stopped with a Bi-Est dose of "1 and 2 drops." If, however, she is still not sleeping optimally, she can increase her progesterone by 1 drop every seven nights until she awakens in the morning with symptoms of progesterone overdose. An example of this would be feeling a bit groggy as if she had taken a slight overdose of a sleeping pill the night before. From that point on, she reduces her nighttime dose back to where she no longer awakens in the morning with symptoms of progesterone excess.

We have discovered through experience and testing that a good limit for the amount of progesterone applied per application is 6 drops. Here are the reasons why:

- 6 drops of oil is a nice and not too excessive amount of oil to apply at any one time: beyond 6 drops, the skin can get a bit too oily.

- Notice the mg/ml difference between Bi-Est 30 mg/ml and progesterone 200 mg/ml. The difference in these two most common formulations reflects the greater need for progesterone, milligram for milligram, in a younger woman's body. The highest concentration a pharmacist can use to formulate transdermal progesterone is 200 mg/ml. Otherwise, believe me, we would prescribe a higher dosage. Thus, absorbing an optimal amount of progesterone can be more challenging than it is to absorb an optimal amount of Bi-Est. It is actually the younger women with healthier and more hydrated skin that tend to absorb progesterone more successfully. Ultimately, this will be discovered by 24-hour urine hormone testing. Through close inspection of hundreds of my patients' hormone test results over the years, I have discovered that most women who are able to absorb transdermal progesterone will most commonly do so by using up to

6 drops. If it takes more than 6 drops, there is usually a skin absorption challenge. At that point, I will switch to an oral micronized compounded progesterone. I'll describe this in an upcoming chapter.

Recall that progesterone is a great "calmer." Lack of sufficient progesterone can lead to a type of sleep disturbance that is different from that of the sleep disturbance caused by an estrogen deficiency. As you may have experienced, an estrogen deficiency often triggers a hot flash which can be accompanied by a surge of adrenaline. This is quite disturbing in the middle of the night. Once again, because of the particular sleep benefit that progesterone provides, and since we are not concerned with "spiking," most women take their progesterone only at bedtime. Beyond the basic sleep advantage of progesterone, oral progesterone compounded in capsules can provide an additional special benefit for assisting with sleep for a reason that relates to how it is biochemically processed.

As I have mentioned, some women will also take their progesterone in the morning along with their Bi-Est. These women do not get sleepy from that morning progesterone dose. They often report that it assists them with having a calm mood during the day and that they like to balance their Bi-Est with progesterone each time they apply their hormones.

*Titration involves finding your optimal dosages clinically by starting with lowish dosages and gradually increasing over time until you alleviate the symptoms of insufficiency. All the while, you stay shy of or back down from symptoms of hormonal excess.*

*Converting from One Type of Hormone Treatment to Another*

Many women have made the change from one type of hormone replacement therapy and dosage to another. The most common examples include:

- Changing from an oral estrogen, such as Premarin or Prempro to bio-identical transdermal estrogens.
- Changing from estradiol in a patch to compounded estrogens in a gel, cream, or organic oils base.
- Changing from compounded estrogens in a gel or cream base to an organic oils base.

My favorite process for any of the above conversions is always the same:

- The first step includes a customary, comprehensive new patient evaluation along with the prescribing of Bi-Est 30 mg/ml and progesterone 200 mg/ml.
- Once my patient receives the new hormones that I have prescribed, she is to stop taking all of the hormones she had been taking.
- At the first hint of an estrogen deficiency symptom (insufficient estrogen is usually the first to cause deficiency symptoms), I ask her to begin the protocol that I have recommended (see earlier pages of this chapter).
- Thus, she begins the dose determination process through titration, including that of testosterone and DHEA, if needed.

This process is very straightforward and reliable most of the time. However, at times, there can be a few transition challenges that you and your healthcare professional can work through. (If a practitioner is prescribing the organic oils, if and when they desire, they can always consult with me.)

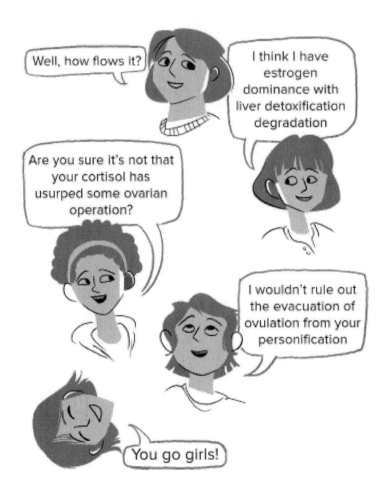

Chapter Nine

# Application Sites and Methods

*Where and How*

So far, we've covered a number of important topics:

- We've placed our initial focus on progesterone and estrogen.

- We've introduced you to "titration": the process of starting with a low dose and gradually increasing the dose until the symptoms of insufficiency are alleviated. Should the dose titration increase to the point that symptoms of excess occur, back down the dose until those symptoms of excess disappear.

- We've told you about when to apply Bi-Est (twice daily) and progesterone (usually, but not always, at bedtime only).

Now, we'd like to show you where and how to apply transdermal hormones and provide additional information regarding when to use them. You can visit our website to view videos on this topic: www.menopausemethod.com.

You've now heard about Bi-Est. The proper routes of Bi-Est administration are to the skin or mucous membranes: transdermal, external transperianal mucosa, and under special circumstances, translabial and transvaginal. Though the sublingual route is possible, it has drawbacks and is not something I recommend or prescribe. Oral administration of estrogens, as discussed previously, are to be avoided.

Let's begin our discussion with what I have found to be the most common and successful route, which is to rub the hormones into your skin or mucous membranes. Many substances absorb very well through the skin. Bi-Est is surely one of them. Though it will absorb from any area of the skin, absorption will vary depending upon the location. For example, absorption from the soft skin of the forearm will be much better than from the thicker skin on the soles of your feet!

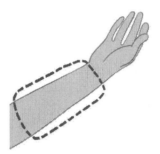

I suggest that you begin application of Bi-Est to the soft skin of the forearm as this is one of the most absorptive areas of skin on your body. However, this will not be the only area where Bi-Est is applied. If you were to rub Bi-Est into only one area, eventually the skin could become oversaturated and absorption could diminish. Therefore, after an initial treatment program is well underway, we begin to rotate the sites of application.

There are specific instructions associated with each area of the skin. I recommend reserving the inner forearms as the location exclusively for the application of Bi-Est. Thus, you would ordinarily *not* apply other hormones to that area. Likewise, for other areas of your body. For example, if you are applying progesterone to your inner thighs, I suggest that you keep the inner thigh area exclusively for the use of progesterone.

Other areas that I recommend you include when rotating Bi-Est are the lateral thighs and possibly the buttocks. There is one special exception regarding the buttocks: if you are sharing a toilet seat with anyone, you need to avoid applying Bi-Est to the toilet seat area of the buttocks. If you were to apply hormones to that area, immediately sit on a toilet seat, and someone else were to sit on that toilet seat immediately or soon after you, they would receive a dose of the hormones.

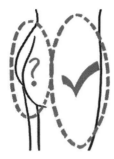 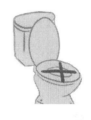

The outer arm, outer forearm, and deltoid region of the shoulder also work well for Bi-Est.

Though the inner arms have soft skin and are a site that can absorb hormones well, we recommend that you do not apply Bi-Est to this location. This is because of the close proximity between the inner arm and the breast; consequently, there is the possibility of transmission of Bi-Est to the breast by direct contact. This site *can* be a good location for progesterone, as transmission of progesterone to the breast is not a concern in most cases.

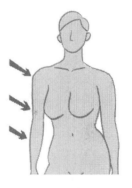

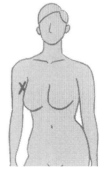

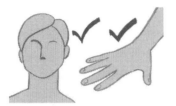

Women have taught me about the refinement of the application of Bi-Est and progesterone: they place either of the hormones onto their hands, rub their hands lightly together, then rub the hormone into one of the recommended areas of the body. They refrain from rubbing all of these hormones into the chosen site, saving a small amount of residual hormone on their hands. Next, they rub that residual into their face, neck, and the back of their hands. Many women do this daily regardless of where they are applying their hormones. This is because the face, neck, and back of the hands are the most vulnerable areas of the skin to sun exposure. Estrogens and progesterone are excellent and restorative for the skin.

There are areas besides the inner arm where we do not want you to apply Bi-Est. Once again, we do not want the direct estrogenic stimulation of breast glandular tissue. Therefore, you should avoid applying estrogen to your

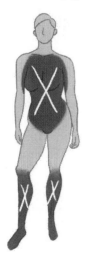 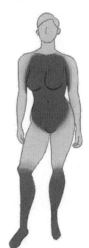

breasts or near your breasts. Thus, we suggest that you do not apply estrogen to the area below the neck to above the pubic bone and the area between the shoulders. And lastly, that you avoid application below the knees because of the possible vulnerability of the dependent leg veins. Medical experience with birth control pills has taught us something about this vulnerability.

We also recommend an occasional application to the soles of your feet. This is not for any absorption you may or may not receive but for the health of the skin of your soles.

Regarding facial skin, many compounding pharmacies often prepare special formulations that contain estriol along with other specialized ingredients that are designed specifically for application to the face. In fact, some pharmacists are experts in creating preparations for the restoration and health of the facial skin. The women in my practice who are using these formulations extol their virtues!

The illustrations below show where to apply progesterone. One favorite location, and the initial location that I most often suggest for the application of transdermal progesterone, is the inner thighs. When the time comes to begin rotating progesterone sites (in one month or two), the

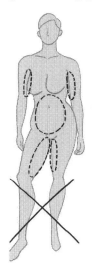 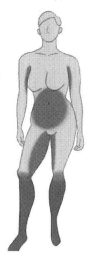

abdomen is a good place to include. Again, the inner arms are also fine for progesterone. There are a certain number of women with fibrocystic breasts who experience relief and healing over time when progesterone is applied directly to the breasts. I refrained from illustrating this in the figures as some women will experience breast tenderness when applying progesterone directly to this area. I recommend that you talk to your health professional if you wish to consider applying progesterone directly to your breasts. Again, with progesterone, I advise that you do not apply it to the area below your knees as these areas have vulnerable veins. Some women have developed phlebitis when taking birth control pills—all of which have artificial progesterone in them.

Along the way, you have learned that transdermally applied hormones can transmit to loved ones. We have conducted testing[9.1] to look more closely at the possibility of transmission, and we have discovered some facts about it, such as:

1. Hormones in oils, gels, and creams absorb well and quickly into the skin of most women.

2. We recommend rubbing these hormones in vigorously. For example, if you put 2 drops of oil onto the soft skin of your forearms and rub your forearms together vigorously, you will feel your skin become warm and notice that within a short period of time your skin will feel quite dry. This occurs for so many women.

3. Approximately 1/2 hour after "rub-in" time, 95% of the hormones you have applied will have absorbed. If you were to wash that area at that time, with minimal washing, there would be *no* residual hormone remaining to transmit to anyone.

4. If you are using transdermal progesterone, we suggest that you reserve the inner thigh area for this hormone and that you do not use the inner thighs for the application of Bi-Est. Progesterone transmission to a loved one, as in intimate contact, would not be of consequence.

5. If you were to transmit freshly applied hormones to anyone and that person washed the area right away, any transmission would become insignificant.

IMPORTANT: I would like you to know that it is not my

> intent to give you unnecessary concern. For example, I caution you not to apply Bi-Est to your inner arm, so there will be no transferring of this hormone to the breast. But, should you happen to rub your arm against your breast and transmit Bi-Est, it is of no significance or concern. You could wash it off, or not, and it would not be a big deal. Would it be a big deal if you rubbed Bi-Est directly into your breast skin every day for 10 years? Maybe yes, maybe no. However, our overall approach is to pay attention to the details to the greatest extent possible to make this process as safe and elegant as can be. You will find this everywhere in our method.

*When to Apply Hormones During the Month*
I have already described the twice-daily application of Bi-Est and the nighttime application of progesterone. I have also mentioned there are exceptions regarding progesterone. Some women like to apply an additional dose of progesterone in the mornings as well, as it contributes a calming effect to daytime mood.

Summary of Bi-Est and Progesterone
Optimal Application Sites

Bi-Est                                   Progesterone

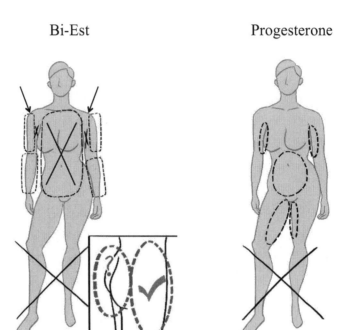

*Stopping Hormones Once a Month*

Now, I would like to explain *when* in the month to use Bi-Est and progesterone. Any woman taking these hormones should take a break from using them once a month. To understand this approach, let's refer to the basic model of this regime: the normal menstrual cycle. Estrogen and progesterone levels are depicted in Figure 9a on the following page. Note that, as day 28 of the cycle approaches, there is dramatic decline in both of these hormone levels. It is this cascade of the hormones that triggers menstruation in a young woman.

Also, note that, on days 1–5 (during menstruation), both estrogen and progesterone levels remain very low. Thus, once a month, a young woman's estrogen and progesterone levels fall to very low amounts comparatively. And, as you can see, progesterone levels are robust only in the second half (luteal phase) of the cycle (and only if a woman ovulates!).

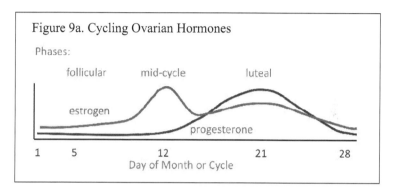

Figure 9a. Cycling Ovarian Hormones

Phases:

follicular          mid-cycle          luteal

estrogen

progesterone

1      5                12            21              28
Day of Month or Cycle

## *Progesterone Rx During Perimenopause*

Our hormonal treatment programs derive somewhat from the pattern of the female menstrual cycle. Regarding progesterone treatment during *perimenopause,* let's consider a woman who is still menstruating yet is having symptoms and signs of progesterone decline, or outright deficiency (see the symptoms of progesterone deficiency on page 79 and in the appendix). We would begin to augment progesterone just prior to mid-cycle and continue it through day 28, or the onset of menstruation.

The exact day to start progesterone in a menstrual month and the amount of progesterone to use is best based on symptom alleviation, as described in Chapter Eight: Hormone Dose Determination. During perimenopause, it is important to stop the administration of progesterone just prior to the anticipated onset of menses.

> When I began working earnestly with women in menopause over two decades ago, I was learning right along with them about how best to accomplish this entire process and often relied significantly on their input. I remember suggesting to Andrea S., who was still menstruating, yet experiencing significant progesterone insufficiency symptoms (and obviously not ovulating) that she should "copy Nature" and use progesterone from days 14–28. In a few months' time, she called and said, "This progesterone is great. I feel like myself again... that is, on days 14–28 of my cycle when I am taking the progesterone. I stop it on day 29 and do okay for another week. But, by day 7 of the new cycle, I strongly feel that I need progesterone again. Why can't I begin taking it on day 6?" I clearly remember that I smiled and said, "Sure, go right ahead." I was well aware that Andrea felt this from the inside and knew best what was right for her body. In addition, once Nature stops producing ovarian progesterone, our attempts to copy Nature by supplying a transdermal progesterone are going to be at best, trials. I opt for what feels best to my patients and confirm by testing and monitoring.

So many women have an internal feel about the optimal time to resume their progesterone. Some stay with the days of 14–28. Most women in my practice start it earlier and use it from days 7–28. Some women start it as soon as they resume their estrogen. And, there are those who are so sensitive to progesterone that they take it intermittently during the month, only when it feels right for them to do so.

*Progesterone Rx During Menopause*

When administering progesterone to a woman in menopause, I recommend one of the three following approaches:

- Stop progesterone on day one of the new calendar month (this will be the same day that you stop Bi-Est), and resume progesterone on the same day that you resume Bi-Est. You will learn how to determine the restarting day for Bi-Est in the upcoming pages. *This is the most common method, as most women ultimately feel best with this approach.*

- Or, stop progesterone on day one of the new calendar month, and resume progesterone on day 12 of the month.

- Or, stop progesterone on day one of the new calendar month, and resume progesterone on day seven of the month.

Once again, ideally, the choice of methods one, two, or three above (or minor variations thereof), plus the amount of progesterone used are optimally chosen based on the principles of titration. Dosages determined should be adequate to alleviate the symptoms of insufficiency while falling shy of or backing down from the symptoms of excess. Likewise, the monthly timing of progesterone treatment is also determined by "feel." Ultimately, the dosages are confirmed by hormone testing, along with monitoring of the breasts, bones, and uterine lining.

*Bi-Est Rx During Perimenopause*

Now, we will look at the case of a *perimenopausal* woman who is still menstruating yet showing symptoms and signs of estrogen decline. Once again, titration is the key to dose determination and timing. In this situation, the ovary is still producing significant amounts of estrogen. Therefore, you will be augmenting the estrogens that are still being produced. Although the amount of estrogens produced in this case have declined enough to produce symptoms of estrogen deficiency such as hot flashes, for example, there is still sufficient ovarian estrogen production for a woman to menstruate. For this reason, augmentation of estrogens with transdermal Bi-Est during perimenopause will be with minimal amounts, if at all.

### Bi-Est Rx During Menopause

When a woman is in menopause, the dose determination of Bi-Est is achieved by titration and always ultimately confirmed by 24-hour urine hormone testing. As far as *when* to administer during the month, I generally recommend that you cease treatment on day one of each calendar month. Next, I will describe the method by which to determine the day to resume treatment.

### Stopping Hormones Once a Month and When to Resume

Once again, I would like to elaborate on stopping hormones once a month and when to resume treatment. We want to mimic the monthly cascade to low hormone levels that take place in a young cycling woman. This is a safeguard to prevent long-term hormone accumulation in the body fat from these fat-soluble hormones if daily dosages were to be slightly higher than optimal.

How long do we stop hormones each month? We have each woman determine her own dosing schedule. I recommend the following process:

- Stop hormones for one, two, three, or four days (and possibly longer) once each month on the first calendar day of the month. The day to resume is determined by the first time a symptom of hormone insufficiency occurs. Let's say, for example, that on days one and two of stoppage a woman feels fine and does not develop any symptoms of estrogen deficiency. Then, for instance, on day 3 she feels a "warm rush." Mission accomplished! That warm rush tells us that her hormone levels fell so low as to cause a symptom of deficiency.

- From that time on, and for all subsequent months, she would only omit her hormones for two days instead of three and then resume treatment on day 3 of stoppage; in this example, it will be on the third day of the month. This will allow hormone levels to fall each month but should prevent the warm rush from occurring. A warm rush is not necessary each month. We do not need hormone levels to drop too low, only to a reasonable low. Although a menstruating woman has a major fall in her estrogen and progesterone levels each month prior to and during her period, her levels do not fall so low as to cause a warm rush!

## *To Summarize and Elaborate*

Let's review when to take hormones during the month:

- Apply Bi-Est approximately 28 days per month, plus or minus, then stop. A simple way to remember this is to stop all hormones on the first calendar day of each month and resume on the day you have determined (one day prior to the day that symptoms occurred).

- There are three options regarding the monthly timing for progesterone:
  - Begin and end on the same day as estrogens (this is by far the most common approach).
  - Begin on day 14, and stop on the first day of each month.
  - Choose any starting day that feels best to you, and stop on the first day of each month.
- Dosages of Bi-Est and progesterone remain constant each day they are taken.
- Bi-Est is taken twice daily, and progesterone is usually taken at bedtime only—though some women do add a second dose of progesterone in the morning.
- Some women prefer to stop their hormones on the full moon, others on the new moon, others near the end of the month. You choose what feels best to you. Whenever you stop, resumption should occur as described above, one day less than the number of days it took for symptoms to resume after stopping hormones.

There are recurring themes and goals in my menopause practice:

- Help women learn as much as possible and, with best case scenario, sense how they are feeling from each hormone they are using
- Provide guidelines for appropriate dosages and assist with overall regimens
- Assist women as they titrate to optimal dosages
- Confirm hormone levels are optimal by 24-hour urine hormone testing

Interestingly, by the time of hormone testing, many women will have arrived at optimal or near optimal hormone levels. So often they develop an internal feel for the hormones and their own needs, and thus arrive at their optimal regimens "clinically" based on "sensing" their own bodies.We then confirm with testing and often see that hormone levels are optimal or require a minor tweaking of the dosages. This system, with few exceptions, works great! Having said that, of great importance is the fact that testing occasionally reveals that a woman has titrated up to excessive dosages and did not feel it! We always do the 24-hour urine hormone test! By defining the optimal number of drops of each hormone and supplying just over a one-month supply of the organic oils/hormone mixture (8.5 ml per bottle), we have built in another safeguard against overdose. Thus, if a woman runs out of hormones before a month has elapsed, her practitioner will know, and she will understand that she has exceeded her prescribed amount of optimal drops per day. These optimal dosages turn out to be:

- Bi-Est: 2 drops in the morning, 3 drops in the evening; and

- Progesterone: a maximum of 6 drops at bedtime.

*Steady Dosing vs Variation in Dosing...*
*plus General Levels of Hormone Dosages*

To be clear, I *am* an advocate of:

- steady daily dosing; and

- stopping Bi-Est and progesterone for a few days each month.

### I am <u>not</u> an advocate of ...

- varying the dosages throughout the month to mimic the pattern of the menstrual cycle;

- restoring youthful hormone levels; and

- maintaining or bringing back a menstrual period.

Shouldn't we be more precise about following the exact pattern of the "menstrual hormonal curves" (see Figure 9a) in treating women in menopause and, as such, vary the dosages day to day? Well, one hallmark of those curves is that the hormone levels plummet at the end of each cycle and remain low during menstruation. Thus, by stopping hormonal treatment in a menopausal woman once a month, we are honoring that decline in hormones. This is one aspect of "cycling." However, from there on, I diverge from modeling a young woman's cycle.

As I mentioned, I am not a proponent of maintaining or restoring menstrual cycles. For one thing, it requires robust and, ultimately, supra-physiologic levels of estrogen dosages to accomplish this in a menopausal woman. *Often, it requires approximately 3 to 10 times the already rich levels of estrogen found in a younger woman.* This may come as a surprise. Why wouldn't it merely require the usual hormone levels that a woman had in her past to sustain or restore a menstrual period? Well, I don't have an explanation for why this is so... it just is! I found this out by serendipitously testing women who came to me on a "sustain or restore the period" hormone treatment regimen, which is being advocated and implemented by some practitioners. I immediately noted that their estradiol and progesterone *dosages* were exceedingly high in comparison to common menopausal treatment dosages. Before having these new patients discontinue their regimens, I performed 24-hour urine hormone tests on them. I suspected urinary hormone levels were going to be very, very high... and they were. I have also had discussions and reviewed the results with the director of a hormone lab. He corroborated my results with the results of other women on this regimen who were tested through his lab. It is important to know that it takes far higher levels of estrogen to sustain or restore a menstrual period in a woman of menopausal age than it does in a young woman—3 to 8 times the upper limit of normal hormone levels appear on testing!

I am a major devotee of the medical, scientific literature and am deeply familiar with it regarding menopause, hormones, and risks. Although the final answers are not yet in, I do have strong opinions.

First of all, I am a firm believer in treating most women in menopause—and treating them with bio-identical hormones. For most women, the important benefits far outweigh the risks.[9.2] Without a doubt, the risk of developing significant health problems as the result of *no* treatment are very substantial.

Secondly, it doesn't take much! Lowish dosages of estrogen are sufficient to alleviate symptoms and support the health of most crucial estrogen-related health issues (e.g., the vagina, bones, brain, arteries, bladder, etc.). These dosages produce hormone levels on testing that are most often quite a bit lower than those found in young menstruating women. In my training seminars for health professionals, www.menopausemethod.com, I define in precise detail the optimal dosage and testing levels. Basically, I am a "low-dose guy." In my opinion, low dosages (not too low) work very well to confer almost all important benefits while minimizing risks.

Third (we've touched upon this earlier), regards the variable-dose approach. So, why not design a treatment program that more precisely mimics the "menstrual curves" (Figure 9a earlier in this chapter)? A decade ago, I was curious about "copying Nature" and, being a lover of math and spreadsheets, I set out to do just that. First, I studied how much total estrogen and progesterone individual patients of mine were using each month (having discovered this through titration and testing while the patients were using steady dosing levels). Then, I discovered a way to recalculate the daily dosages so they would precisely mimic the curves. The dosages were different almost every day. And, over the course of a month, the total amount of Bi-Est used equaled the amount a patient was taking when they were using constant daily dosages. Many of my patients tried this method. Interestingly enough, it just did not work out as planned. A colleague of mine and I decided to test two women who were on the new regimen at three different times during their cycles: days 7, 12, and 21. Instead of seeing 24-hour urine hormone test results that mimicked the curves, our lowest numbers were on day 7, our middle values were on day 12, and our highest hormone values were on day 21! Because the dosing followed the curves, theoretically the highest values should have been when the dosages were highest, on day 12. We attributed these unexpected results, which were different from the pattern of the female cycle, to probable differences in hormones coming directly from the ovary versus those absorbed transdermally. Whatever the actual reasons were, this was enough for me to discontinue this method. Equally, if not even more interesting, was that although copying the dosage pattern of the curves made sense to me, and to many of my female patients who eagerly tried it; over time and one by one, they abandoned this method. On their own, they went back to and preferred steady daily dosages! So much for that theory!

In retrospect, we do not know what copying Nature is for a woman in menopause. If we were to truly copy Nature, we would not administer hormones, as the ovaries are no longer functioning. However, there are too many adverse consequences probable from that approach.

And lastly, there are health professionals trained in specific methods of treating women in menopause that incorporate the administration of hormones in a pattern that replicates the female cycle. In my onion, the main problem with this method is *not* the replication of the phases of the female cycle through a variation in daily dosages. The problem is that the dosages prescribed are 3 to 10 times the levels that are most common in my medical practice and those commonly used by thousands of doctors. Reasons for using high dosages are given by the promulgators of this regimen. A personal communication was once made to me: "It takes higher levels of estrogen to keep a period going or restore one that has ceased!"

I am not at all reassured by this explanation. My understanding, which is derived from the medical literature, is clearly to avoid supra-physiologic levels of hormones.[9.3] I do want to give you my best opinion: I strongly disagree with the method of using high dosages. I am a proponent of minimal amounts of treatment dosages, yet, sufficient to protect organs and alleviate symptoms of insufficiency. Medical studies clearly show the hormone treatment levels required to accomplish this are quite low, as compared to young women. Interestingly enough, levels sufficient to protect or restore the health of the vagina are sufficient to promote the health of the bones and most other estrogen-dependent issues, and again, comparatively, these levels are quite low.[9.4] It just doesn't take much to make a wonderful difference!

There is one exception to prescribing lowish dosages that can occur when treating women with declining cognitive abilities, or even heading towards or already in the dementia spectrum. In a certain number of women, richer than usual dosages of estrogen can help significantly in restoring or maintaining mental function, especially when coupled by a multi-faceted functional medicine approach. As an additional note, any woman with a serious cognitive decline that is not markedly restored with additional estrogen should, in my opinion, seek functional medicine treatment to assess the multiple causatives and often addressable factors.[9.5]

### *"Dermal fatigue" and Other Possible Locations to Apply Bi-Est and Progesterone*

Thus far, I have recommended applying Bi-Est and progesterone to the skin. There are a certain percentage of women who apply hormones to the same area of the skin, year after year, and do fine. However, some women develop transdermal absorption issues. In the ongoing monitoring of women, approximately every one to two years, we repeat the 24-hour urine hormone test, among other evaluations. We can identify a woman who is developing absorption issues from her story of symptom(s) recurrence and/or from her hormone test results. If hormone levels show a decline from one test to the next, even in the face of hormone dosages remaining constant or increasing over time, we know that something is occurring to cause that decline. It could be an issue of diminishing absorption from the area of the skin that is receiving the hormones. This has been called "dermal fatigue."[9,6] It can be the result of a specific area of the skin and the fat beneath it (subcutaneous fat) becoming oversaturated from hormone absorption and, therefore, needing a "break."

One remedy for this is to rotate the absorption sites. Another option can be to utilize a different route of administration. Absorption from mucosal surfaces can be an excellent alternative and can result in higher hormone levels per dose than transdermal administration. Additional locations to utilize include the:

- external part (not inside) of the anus, the "external perianal mucosa";
- inner or outer aspects of the inner vaginal labia ("lips") (for those not having intercourse); and
- inside of the vagina ("intravaginal") (again, for those not having intercourse).

As with all things, there are pros and cons with each location.

Applying hormones to the external perianal mucosa (the external area surrounding the anal orifice, approximately 1/2–3/4 inches in diameter) is an excellent absorptive surface and can be used to remedy dermal fatigue. The optimal time to apply hormones in this location is right after a shower.

Although in or near the vagina can be a location where absorption is very good, there are challenges with these locations. As an example, if a woman is having intercourse, there is a high probability of transmitting hormones to her partner.

As I mentioned previously, we performed a study[9.7] to determine how long a transdermal hormone preparation lingered on the skin after application. We concluded that in 1/2 hour, 95% of the hormones were absorbed, and by 1.5 hours, only a negligible amount was present. Since skin hormone residual disappeared efficiently, I assumed that hormones applied to the intravaginal mucosa would disappear even more rapidly. This proved not to be the case as revealed by the testing of one of my patients. Her vaginal estriol was present 60 hours after application ceased.

This is a "case of one," which means it is not conclusive. More studies need to be done regarding the lingering effects of intravaginally applied Bi-Est and the possibility of transmission during intercourse. For now, I advise women who are having intercourse not to apply Bi-Est intravaginally or to the vaginal labia ("lips").

Also to be considered with labial or vaginal application is the possibility of interfering with the results of the 24-hour urine hormone test. Hormones that are applied in the vagina or on the labia could linger where applied.[9.7] Urine can "wash" over the internal aspect of the internal vaginal labia and also the vagina. In so doing, the urine could directly collect recently applied hormones and confound the test results. One esteemed colleague, who does favor intravaginal hormone application, has patients change their application site to the external perianal mucosa before and during the 24-hour urine collection.

Taking these issues into account, if a woman is not having intercourse but is having issues with dermal fatigue, application of hormones to the labia and/or vagina can be a good solution. As I just mentioned, testing issues can be reasonably circumvented by changing to the perianal mucosa for five days preceding and during the urine collection. The test results will provide a representative reflection of labial/intravaginal application.

As a final note regarding the route of administration, there are some health professionals who favor sublingual formulations. In this case, hormones are compounded into troches that can be placed under the tongue and absorbed through the sublingual mucosa. At first consideration, this would seem like a good method. This is, after all, an excellent location for medications to absorb into the system. For example, it is the original and preferred location to administer nitroglycerin, which is so useful in types of coronary artery emergencies. Hormones also absorb well from under the tongue.

However, even though there are practitioners who prescribe sublingual hormones, I shy away from this route. Often there is a percentage of the sublingual troche that is swallowed after blending in with the oral saliva. I have emphasized reasons not to administer estrogens orally and will say the same about testosterone. Also, sublingual absorption is rapid. In a short time, estrogen levels will "peak" in the blood. Gradual, slow absorption into the blood is a more beneficial approach.

Never say "never." I do have one patient who does well on sublingual progesterone. Since oral progesterone is not a problem, swallowing some of the sublingual progesterone would be fine.

*A Final Note About Dosages and Testing*

No matter what transdermal hormone preparation you use —organic oils, gels, or creams—and no matter what dosage, strength and ratio (for Bi-Est), the most important thing I want you to remember is that when you have stabilized on your regimen, it is *imperative* that you do the 24-hour urine hormone test. I'll explain more later!

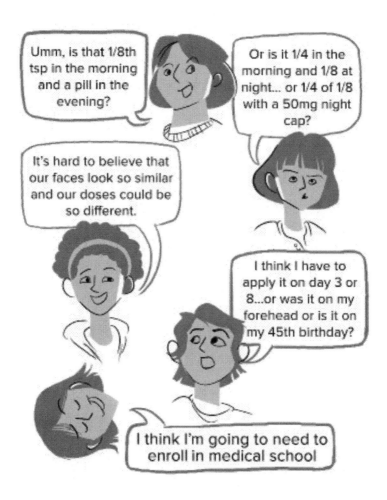

# Chapter Ten

# Formulations:
# The Hormones, Carriers,
# and Dispensing Methods

## *Information Regarding "Carriers"*

I want to address the question, "What's in the jar?" When you receive a prescription for transdermal Bi-Est, progesterone, or testosterone from your compounding pharmacy, the hormones are not the only ingredient in the container. Most often, the hormones are *dissolved* in something called a "carrier" or "base" or "vehicle."

In order to obtain a uniform dispersion (referred to as a "solution") of the hormones and, consequently, yield a constant daily dose from the first dose all the way through to the very last, the hormones must be dissolved in a carrier. That carrier has to be a special type of strong "solvent" capable of dissolving fat because the ovarian hormones are fat-soluble only, and poorly so. They do not dissolve in water. Alcohol is one of those solvents strong enough to dissolve ovarian hormones, and there are many others. Therefore, if the hormones were not dissolved in a carrier, they would not stay evenly dispersed and would settle out to the bottom of the container (Figure 10a). It all makes sense—dissolving the hormones allows for even

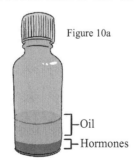

Figure 10a

Oil

Hormones

distribution throughout the container. As a result, each time a woman measures out her dose, she is sure to receive the identical amount of hormone.

There is another reason for the carriers: the hormones that are present in a container are measured in milligrams (mg)—an amount so tiny you would not be able to measure it out if it were not in a carrier. For this reason alone, the hormones need to be placed in a carrier to ensure that your dose of hormone-plus-carrier is measurable in "drops" or milliliters (ml) or fractions of a teaspoon, rather than in amounts too tiny to measure.

In actual practice, it turns out that most of what you are applying to your skin is the carrier. Let's do the math on a common transdermal gel formulation: Bi-Est 2.5 mg/ml. This signifies 2.5 mg (milligrams) of Bi-Est dissolved in 1 ml (milliliter) of the carrier. Therefore, 1 ml contains:

- 2.5 mg of Bi-Est, plus
- 1 ml of the carrier
  - 1 ml of the carrier weighs 1 gram, which = 1000 mg
  - Thus, in 1 ml of Bi-Est 2.5 mg/ml, there are 2.5 mg of Bi-Est and 997.5 mg of the carrier
- Consequently, there is 400 times more carrier than hormone (997.5 ÷ 2.5)
  - Hormone content is 0.25% of the container (2.5 ÷ 1000 x 100)
  - Carrier content is 99.7% (100% - 0.25%) of the container
- Wow!

Patients on Bi-Est gel or cream formulations use approximately one-half milliliter twice daily, applied in divided doses; thus, a total of one milliliter per day. This is a very practical amount of gel to rub onto the skin, not too little and not too much. The amount of Bi-Est in that one milliliter (total daily dose), volume-wise, compares to that of one grain of sand.

So, dissolving ovarian hormones in a carrier solvent sure makes sense and sounds good. Yet, how good is it? Ten years into treating women in menopause, I opened a jar of one of the common compounded prescriptions containing hormone plus carrier that I was using at the time, Bi-Est in a gel base called "Carbopol®." "Hmm," I thought, "This obviously smells of alcohol, at the very least. Hmmm. I have been suggesting that women rub this into their skin twice daily for all of these years. Hmmm. What actually is Carbopol and how "good" is it, I wonder... ?"

Carbopol, which is technically a "polyacrylic acid," is an example of one of the several common solvent carriers used by compounding pharmacists. They have several other choices to offer, such as Lipoderm®, Versabase®, Pluronic Lecithin Organogel (PLO), and others. No matter what carrier we are talking about, they are solvents, or they contain solvents. Again, because ovarian hormones are "poorly soluble," the solvents need to be potent and present in a significant quantity for the ovarian hormones to actually dissolve. As another example, 100 milligrams of progesterone is the maximum amount you can dissolve in one milliliter of Carbopol. Thus, in one milliliter of progesterone-in-Carbopol, 100 milligrams are progesterone, and 900 milligrams are Carbopol. Again, the majority of what a woman is applying is the carrier. My point: what that carrier is made out of matters.

Carbopol has been around for a long time. Over a decade ago, when pharmaceutical manufacturers started responding to the widespread fear of Premarin, knowing full well that there was a market for transdermal bio-identical hormones, they began manufacturing estradiol as a transdermal gel. The most popular of these products, and there are several of them, are in a Carbopol base.

When I had my "aha" moment regarding the odor of solvents, I began researching the nature of the solvents being used. You can turn to the reference section to learn more: it's not a pretty picture.[10.1] The toxic profiles of some of these carrier substances are substantial. As a holistic physician, I am cognizant of toxic exposure in general, as the multitude of toxins that we are exposed to in this modern world have affected every one of us... and some worse than others, especially the sensitive ones amongst us.

A colleague of mine and I began thinking about options. Ultimately, through a friend, I connected with Candace Newman, the "oil lady," who is an expert in essential oils.[10.2] She referred me to wonderful sources. We developed a 100% organic oils blend, the ingredients of which are known to benefit the skin. One of the principle oils we are using has been studied thoroughly as a possible food source by the Nestlé company and passed with flying colors. It has long been a preferred choice by massage therapists. The other two oils, Oenothera (evening primrose) and borage are used as nutritional supplements when taken orally.

For over 10 years, we have been using the organic oils hormone preparations. We have tested hundreds of women using the 24-hour urine hormone test, and the dosages used have correlated with the hormone levels in these patients. The majority of women I treat like or love these oils.

Because we do not include solvents in the organic oils mixture,
the bottles containing the hormones
must be shaken vigorously before
each use, as the contents are a "suspension." This means that the hormones are "suspended" in the oils
mix. After the mixture is thoroughly

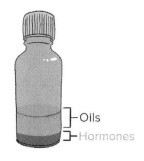

shaken, the hormones will be evenly distributed throughout;
yet, after standing for a while, the oils will float to the top,
and the hormones will settle to the bottom, as shown above.
At one point, early in the development of these formulations,
a colleague of mine with a chemistry and pharmacy background suggested that we add solvents to the oils to bring the
hormones into a uniform solution. Of course, we declined as
that would nullify one of the major benefits.

It is interesting to note that, at one point, we sent out a
bottle of the Bi-Est that was nearly emptied to the bottom—
very little hormones/oil remained—to a reference lab. The
test results showed that what remained in the bottom of the
bottle had a concentration identical to the original concentration that was on the label of the bottle, demonstrating
that shaking the contents into a suspension works. The dosage remains constant, whether the bottle is new or almost
empty. These organic oils-based hormones are prepared in
a 30-milliliter bottle containing 8.5 milliliters, which is a
one-month supply. The bottle is filled one-quarter full for
the purpose of providing ample room to "shake, shake,
shake" the bottle before each use.

In my medical practice, roughly 98% percent of the
transdermal ovarian hormones that I prescribe are in these
organic oils. My other patients need or prefer Carbopol or

other carriers for various reasons. There is no one solution for all women. A practitioner needs to have several tools in working with transdermal and transmucosal hormones.

As a final note on non-oils-based formulations, I mentioned earlier that pharmaceutical manufacturers had developed transdermal estradiol products. These products fall considerably shy of what I would recommend. For one thing, estriol is not included as one of the estrogens. For all that we know about estrogen receptor site beta (ERβ), I always include an abundant amount of estriol in any estrogen prescription. Secondly, as I have mentioned, several of the most popular estradiol transdermal products are prepared in Carbopol. This is no surprise: Carbopol has been in common use for so long in pharmacies. And, as the third issue to me, the manufacturers have chosen to add additional solvents and absorption enhancers to these products. Typical additives are propylene and ethylene glycol and their chemical relatives, among others. These are toxic chemicals and are the main constituents of antifreeze. When I was in my twenties, I used to enjoy working on my cars, even to the point of rebuilding an engine. I never minded the dirt and grease. I did mind emptying my radiator however, as the antifreeze was instantly caustic to my hands, turning my skin a thin crusty white.

When I need an alternative to the oils, which is only rarely, Carbopol itself as the sole carrier is acceptable to me: there are benefits and risks to almost anything in medicine. Carbopol and other carriers routinely used by compounding pharmacists are far more acceptable than the numerous chemicals added to many of the new pharmaceutical gels and patches. Again, 98% of the transdermal hormones I prescribe are in the organic oils mix.

And, the organic oils are, by far, the most preferable to me. There is no toxicity. The organic oils carrier has a direct benefit to the skin. The only downside is the 5 to 8 shakes that are required before opening the bottle each time. For additional information to provide to your doctor, nurse practitioner, or compounding pharmacist about obtaining these oils, you could go to www.menopapusemethod.com and send them the link to the Professionals' page.

*Dispensing Information: Organic Oils, Rx Dosages*

Most all new patients of Menopause Method trained practitioners leave their initial consultation with a prescription for Bi-Est 30 mg/ml 80:20, 8.5 ml (80% estriol, 20% estradiol) as well as a prescription for progesterone 200 mg/ml, 8.5 ml in the organic oils base. (There are a few exceptions, usually early perimenopausal patients receiving just the progesterone Rx and a few early or super-sensitive women receiving a Bi-Est 15 mg/ml Rx.) Over time, a small percentage of patients will need to have aspects of this formulation tweaked (either or both: the mg/ml and/or the percentages of estriol and estradiol).

I start most (but not all) women in menopause on the following protocol ("Most Common Starting Rx"):

1. Bi-Est 30 mg/ml 80:20, 8.5 ml in the organic oils blend

   • 1 drop in the morning plus 1 drop at bedtime (0.4 mgeeq/ drop [see the note in the reference section for an explanation of "mgeeq" [10.3]])

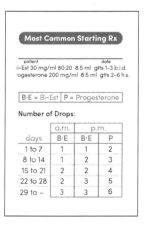

**Most Common Starting Rx**

patient _____ date _____
i-Est 30 mg/ml 80:20  8.5 ml  gtts 1–3 b.i.d.
ogesterone 200 mg/ml  8.5 ml  gtts 2–6 h.s.

B·E = Bi-Est | P = Progesterone

Number of Drops:

| days | a.m. B·E | p.m. B·E | p.m. P |
|---|---|---|---|
| 1 to 7 | 1 | 1 | 2 |
| 8 to 14 | 1 | 2 | 3 |
| 15 to 21 | 2 | 2 | 4 |
| 22 to 28 | 2 | 3 | 5 |
| 29 to – | 3 | 3 | 6 |

- Applied to the soft skin of the inner forearms
- Rubbed in vigorously

2. Progesterone 200 mg/ml, 8.5 ml in the organic oils blend

- 2 drops at bedtime (8.7 mg/drop)
- Applied to the soft skin of the inner thighs
- Rubbed in vigorously

If I suspect a woman has an unusual sensitivity to medications or hormones or has been in menopause for quite a while—let's say longer than a year or, for some, longer than six months—I may start her on 1 drop of Bi-Est in the evening only, along with 1 drop of progesterone. In The Menopause Method, we name this approach the "Lighter Starting Rx." Ordinarily, I would suggest increasing that dose by one drop every seven days if the symptoms of estrogen deficiency were not alleviated by the starting dose. This time we would add that next drop in the morning along with a second drop of progesterone at bedtime.

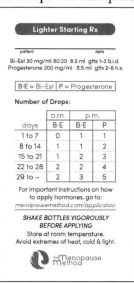

Then, following the directions on the starting dosage titration card, you would continue to titrate up to symptom alleviation while falling shy of or backing down from symptoms of excess. (For more information on titration as well as hormone application, we suggest you view our two videos on these topics, "Getting Your Hormone Dosages Right" and "Hormone Application." Visit www.menopausemethod.com/for-women-in-menopause/getting-started/, and scroll down to the videos.)

When it comes to increasing your estrogen dosage, I advise patience and that you do not yield to the temptation to increase it faster than specified. The longer a woman has been in menopause without hormones, the slower we suggest she increases her dosage. Through the years, many individual adjustments have occurred in her body from hormonal decline. It is a mistake to rush the process of restoration. We want a woman's body to make the readjustments in a kind and patient pace. This may be why patients are called "patients."

For these reasons, there are important issues to consider as a woman is titrating her dosages:

- We set an initial maximum dose of Bi-Est at "3 & 3 drops" (morning and evening). If a woman does not receive full symptom alleviation with this dosage, we have her consult with her provider as this would be a time for further evaluation.

- At times, it seems appropriate to advance treatment at a faster rate than I have mentioned thus far. As we've discussed, progesterone dosages can be increased more rapidly than Bi-Est. Therefore, if sleep has not improved after three to four nights on progesterone, I may recommend increasing the progesterone dose by 1 drop at bedtime. This is especially so when the sleep disturbance is not primarily caused by nocturnal hot flashes, which so often are estrogen deficiency based. Thus, progesterone can be increased by 1 drop twice a week rather than 1 drop once per week. It is important to pay attention to how you are feeling in the morning upon awakening. If you feel unusually groggy, it is probably from excessive progesterone the night before, so back down the dose. Thus, progesterone dosage determination can be a tad more aggressive than the more cautious approach we suggest with Bi-Est.

- I set a maximum dose of progesterone at 6 drops, taken at bedtime. If symptoms of deficiency have not been alleviated, this could call for a change in the dosing method of progesterone to oral administration. Thus, this would be a time to consult with your provider.

- Some women enjoy an additional dose of progesterone in the morning, sufficient to enhance progesterone's benefits, such as calmness or anxiety alleviation. At the same time, staying shy of overdose symptoms, such as daytime grogginess or depression.

- Many women enter menopause and seek treatment for it early on. Their bodies are accustomed to significant levels of hormones. This is especially so for women who were "estrogen rich" their entire lives. These women might find our "Most Common Starting Dosage" regimen a bit lower and slower than optimal. With this in mind, I often will be inclined to begin this patient on richer startup dosages ("Enhanced Starting Rx" card on the right). You will see that the rate of the dose increases for Bi-Est are faster, as are the increased dosages and pace for progesterone.

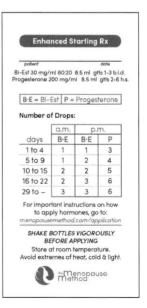

The three different "starting dose cards" show examples of common dosage possibilities. Often enough, individualizing a woman's protocol may call for a special regimen, and so there is a fourth card ("Customized Rx Schedule") to be designed by your practitioner.

No dosing regimen is written in stone. Any of the starting dosages suggested are only guidelines and can quickly be altered as each woman acquires an internal feel for the hormones, symptom alleviation, and the symptoms of excess—all of which play a part in her dose discovery by titration.

Again, we encourage you to visit our website, www.menopausemethod.com/for-women-in-menopause/getting-started/, and scroll down to view the two videos: "Getting Your Hormone Dosages Right" and "Hormone Application."

Your dosage discovery is also supported by the information provided on the "Finding Your Optimal Dose" cards below. Here you will find the symptoms of hormone insufficiency and excess.

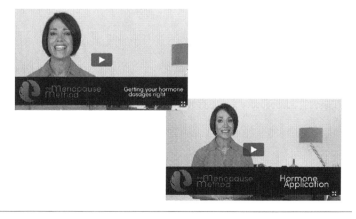

## *Dispensing Methods: Organic Oils, Additional Information*

I would like to begin by showing you an artist's rendition of the bottles containing the organic oils and explain how to dispense the oils from them. Pictured is a 30-milli-

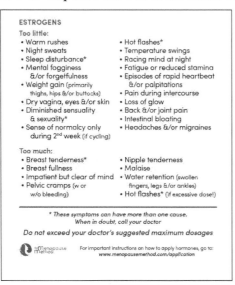

ESTROGENS

Too little:
- Warm rushes
- Night sweats
- Sleep disturbance*
- Mental fogginess &/or forgetfulness
- Weight gain (primarily thighs, hips &/or buttocks)
- Dry vagina, eyes &/or skin
- Diminished sensuality & sexuality*
- Sense of normalcy only during 2nd week (if cycling)
- Hot flashes*
- Temperature swings
- Racing mind at night
- Fatigue or reduced stamina
- Episodes of rapid heartbeat &/or palpitations
- Pain during intercourse
- Loss of glow
- Back &/or joint pain
- Intestinal bloating
- Headaches &/or migraines

Too much:
- Breast tenderness*
- Breast fullness
- Impatient but clear of mind
- Pelvic cramps (w or w/o bleeding)
- Nipple tenderness
- Malaise
- Water retention (swollen fingers, legs &/or ankles)
- Hot flashes* (if excessive dose!)

*These symptoms can have more than one cause.
When in doubt, call your doctor*

*Do not exceed your doctor's suggested maximum dosages*

Menopause Method — For important instructions on how to apply hormones, go to: www.menopausemethod.com/application

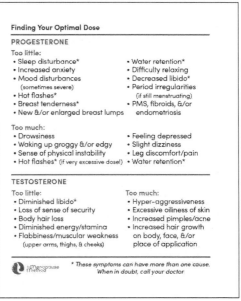

Finding Your Optimal Dose

PROGESTERONE

Too little:
- Sleep disturbance*
- Increased anxiety
- Mood disturbances (sometimes severe)
- Hot flashes*
- Breast tenderness*
- New &/or enlarged breast lumps
- Water retention*
- Difficulty relaxing
- Decreased libido*
- Period irregularities (if still menstruating)
- PMS, fibroids, &/or endometriosis

Too much:
- Drowsiness
- Waking up groggy &/or edgy
- Sense of physical instability
- Hot flashes* (if very excessive dose!)
- Feeling depressed
- Slight dizziness
- Leg discomfort/pain
- Water retention*

TESTOSTERONE

Too little:
- Diminished libido*
- Loss of sense of security
- Body hair loss
- Diminished energy/stamina
- Flabbiness/muscular weakness (upper arms, thighs, & cheeks)

Too much:
- Hyper-aggressiveness
- Excessive oiliness of skin
- Increased pimples/acne
- Increased hair growth on body, face, &/or place of application

Menopause Method — *These symptoms can have more than one cause. When in doubt, call your doctor.*

liter bottle containing 8.5 milliliters of Bi-Est in the organic oils, just over a one-month supply. The bottle is one-quarter full to allow plenty of room to "shake-shake-shake" the bottle (approximately five shakes) before removing the cap. After shaking and removing the cap, turn the bottle completely upside down over your forearm. The first drop may come out slowly, but the ensuing drops come out more rapidly.

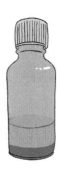

With the formulations prescribed, a bottle should last one month, depending on the number of drops you are using, the strength of the prescription, and the number of days you cease using hormones each month. However, if you exceed 3 drops of Bi-Est twice daily, you will run out of hormones before the

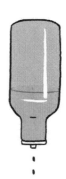

end of the month. This is intentional: the number of drops in each bottle is precisely calculated—it's a built-in safety feature of The Menopause Method. We have looked for and created measures that prevent excessive dosing with estrogens. Ultimately, most women do very well in finding their optimal dose through titration. There are a small but significant number, however, who wind up taking an excessive dose. When this occurs, it is usually because:

- The woman did not feel clear symptoms of overdose and, thus, titration was continued, exceeding optimal levels.

- Absorption was above average, making it easy to overdose unexpectedly.

- 24-hour urine hormone testing was needed earlier than expected to help sort out a challenging case.

- Metabolism or hormone balance issues exist, which require 24-hour urine hormone test results to unveil. These issues call for a special tweak of dosage strength, ratio, or balancing with other hormones.

- Initial dosing instructions were not precisely followed as directed.

- 24-hour urine hormone testing was not done to assess levels once deficiency symptoms were alleviated.

Also to be noted are the women who titrate to what appear to be excessive dosages, yet on 24-hour urine testing are shown to have normal or even below normal estrogen levels. The problem in this case is clearly poor absorption through the skin. This is another example of how imperative it is to do the 24-hour urine hormone test: it is surely not healthy to have insufficient hormone levels for an extended period of time.

Next, let's talk about individualizing your dosage of Bi-Est:

- From the initial Rx of Bi-Est 30 mg/ml 80:20, you are going to discover how many drops are optimal for you. So much is dependent upon your individual needs; your sensitivity to anything you take; your available hormone receptor sites, and of great importance, your absorption. Once you have determined your dose, the optimal number of drops of Bi-Est per day is 2 in the morning and 3 in the evening.

- Commonly, some women will titrate to "2 & 2" drops, others to "2 & 3" drops, and still others to "3 & 3" drops.

- If you titrate to "1 & 2" or "1 & 1," it is likely that the initial Rx is on the strong side for you, or you have exuberant absorption. In either case, should you need to add an extra drop for any reason, such as increased estrogen need at a time of stress, that 1 drop will be more potent than optimal for an incremental increase. Without going into a discussion of potency and mge-eq,[10.3] a decrease in potency of your next prescription will allow for a 1 drop increase that will not be too great of a potency increase. Consequently, any increase in this adjusted dose of 1 drop, up or down, will allow you to titrate with smaller dosages; thus, you will be more likely to make an optimal incremental increase or decrease.

- If this sounds daunting or challenging to understand, no worries. This method is ideally designed to provide the appropriate strength of Bi-Est so that you will average 5 drops per day, provide just over a one-month prescription, and minimize the possibility of an excessive dose of estrogen. This is important. In a careful study of 24-hour urine hormone test results of my patients and those of Menopause Method practitioners, excessive doses of estrogens, though not frequent, are common enough.

- Here's what is most important about these tailored prescription strengths of Bi-Est and the drop count of 5 per day: these formulations provide a built-in high probability that you will not titrate into overdose! For example, if your ideal dose through titration is "3 & 3" drops per day, and provided 24-hour urine hormone testing confirms that estrogens and metabolites are optimal, we can then customize your next Rx by changing the mg/ml (and even the ratio if it needs adjusting as well) to have the final outcome translate into a Bi-Est prescription that provides 5 drops per day.

- *Ultimately, our goal is to achieve optimal symptom relief, support and protection of the bones, brain, vagina, bladder, muscles, etc., along with great lab results and healthy mammograms.*

*Starter Tools*

All patients of the physicians or nurse practitioners that subscribe to The Menopause Method educational program, www.menopausemethod.com, leave their first office visit with the following starter tools:

- Access to our online videos explaining how and where to apply hormones as well as how to determine optimal dosages by titration. Again, you can view these videos at www.menopausemethod.com. (Simply scroll down to the videos.)

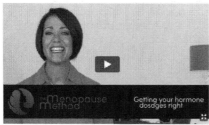

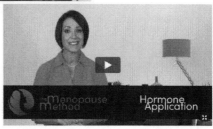

- One of four "Patient Instruction Cards": Most Common Starting Rx, Lighter Starting Rx, Enhanced Starting Rx, or a Customized Rx Schedule. (The Customized Rx Schedule will be designed by your physician, nurse practitioner, or prescribing pharmacist. He/she will base your protocol on his/her medical assessment of your initial needs and sensitivities.)A laminated "Finding Your Optimal Dose" card listing the symptoms of deficiency and excess for each hormone to assist you in dose determination (see the following page).

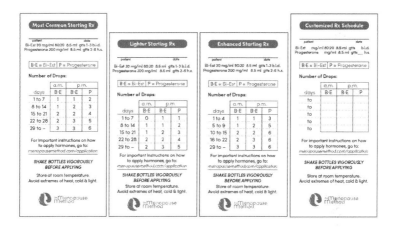

During your first visit with your Menopause Method provider, you will receive your specific dosage recommendations card (one of the four pictured above) that will indicate the starting number of drops of Bi-Est and progesterone, when to apply them, and when to increase your dosage.

For example, a patient is given the Most Common Starting Rx card and, thus, begins on a Bi-Est dosage of 1 drop in the morning and 1 drop at bedtime along with 2 drops of progesterone at bedtime, as depicted on the card

**Finding Your Optimal Dose**

### ESTROGENS

Too little:
- Warm rushes
- Night sweats
- Sleep disturbance*
- Mental fogginess
  &/or forgetfulness
- Weight gain (primarily
  thighs, hips &/or buttocks)
- Dry vagina, eyes &/or skin
- Diminished sensuality
  & sexuality*
- Sense of normalcy only
  during 2nd week (if cycling)

- Hot flashes*
- Temperature swings
- Racing mind at night
- Fatigue or reduced stamina
- Episodes of rapid heartbeat
  &/or palpitations
- Pain during intercourse
- Loss of glow
- Back &/or joint pain
- Intestinal bloating
- Headaches &/or migraines

Too much:
- Breast tenderness*
- Breast fullness
- Impatient but clear of mind
- Pelvic cramps (w or
  w/o bleeding)

- Nipple tenderness
- Malaise
- Water retention (swollen
  fingers, legs &/or ankles)
- Hot flashes* (if excessive dose!)

*These symptoms can have more than one cause.
When in doubt, call your doctor*

*Do not exceed your doctor's suggested maximum dosages*

 the Menopause Method  For important instructions on how to apply hormones, go to:
www.menopausemethod.com/application

---

**Finding Your Optimal Dose**

### ESTROGENS

Too little:
- Warm rushes
- Night sweats
- Sleep disturbance*
- Mental fogginess
  &/or forgetfulness
- Weight gain (primarily
  thighs, hips &/or buttocks)
- Dry vagina, eyes &/or skin
- Diminished sensuality
  & sexuality*
- Sense of normalcy only
  during 2nd week (if cycling)

- Hot flashes*
- Temperature swings
- Racing mind at night
- Fatigue or reduced stamina
- Episodes of rapid heartbeat
  &/or palpitations
- Pain during intercourse
- Loss of glow
- Back &/or joint pain
- Intestinal bloating
- Headaches &/or migraines

Too much:
- Breast tenderness*
- Breast fullness
- Impatient but clear of mind
- Pelvic cramps (w or
  w/o bleeding)

- Nipple tenderness
- Malaise
- Water retention (swollen
  fingers, legs &/or ankles)
- Hot flashes* (if excessive dose!)

*These symptoms can have more than one cause.
When in doubt, call your doctor*

*Do not exceed your doctor's suggested maximum dosages*

 the Menopause Method  For important instructions on how to apply hormones, go to:
www.menopausemethod.com/application

(page 129, next to days "1 to 7"). If all goes well yet some but not all menopausal symptoms are alleviated (as listed on the Finding Your Optimal Dose card):

- This patient would increase the evening dose of Bi-Est to 2 drops during days 8 to 14. At the same time, she would increase her dose of progesterone to 3 drops. We call this "1 & 2 and 3."

- Let's say by day 14 most symptoms are relieved, but not all. She would then increase to "2 & 2 and 4."

- However, if after four days on this regimen she began to develop breast tenderness (a symptom of possible estrogen excess), she would then decrease her dosage back to "1 & 2 and 3."

Many dosing variations are possible. The more experience you have in working with hormones, the better you will be able to fine-tune your protocol. This is one of the major purposes of this book and our method. We believe it is best for you to be an active participant in this process; after all, there are symptoms that only you will feel and know.

For years, we have strived to make this process absolutely as safe, easy, and elegant as possible for patients and their health professionals.

There are many methods and carriers for prescribing and compounding bio-identical hormones. You can enjoy an excellent menopausal treatment program with several different approaches. I have gone into detail about the organic oils base and the accompanying clinical practice materials with the intention of informing all women, including my patients, and the physicians and nurse practitioners who use The Menopause Method.

*Dispensing Methods: Other Carriers and Routes*

*Please note: if you are beginning treatment with The Menopause Method and the organic oils, it will not be necessary for you to read the following section.*

As we discussed earlier, there are other common carriers. Below is an example of a good starting dose for Bi-Est formulated in a gel or cream base:

- Bi-Est in Carbopol, Versabase, or Lipoderm
  2.75 mg/g 73:27 (estriol 2 mg/estradiol 0.75 mg)

  Regarding pump dispensers:

  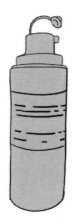

  o There are a variety of pumps. One of the most common delivers 0.5 ml per pump.

  o Thus, if you are using Bi-Est 2.75 mg/ml 73:27, each pump delivers 0.5 mgeeq (see the footnote section[10.3] for an explanation of "mgeeq"). For the experienced practitioner who loves math, the actual strength of the Bi-Est formulation can ultimately be adjusted so that each pump is optimized for the patient. For example, if the concentration is reduced to 2.5 mg/ml 80:20, each pump now delivers 0.4 mgeeq.

  o In a pump bottle, one pump delivers 0.5 ml: one pump twice daily @ 0.5 mgeeq/pump = 1 mgeeq/ two pumps/24 hours.

Occasionally, when a woman has absorption issues and requests Bi-Est in gels or creams, a 5.5 mg/ml (E3 4 mg/E2

1.5 mg) formulation can be prescribed. Thus, with twice the strength, smaller quantities can be applied to the skin. This option is cost efficient as well. Recall, compounding pharmacies usually charge the same amount regardless of the strength and composition of the prescription.

There are other dispensing methods for compounded hormones, such as Bi-Est in a jar. Dosages can be measured out by using special spoons that deliver one-eighth of a teaspoon (0.6 ml) or one-quarter of a teaspoon (1.25 ml). Dosages can also be very accurately determined by loading a 3-milliliter syringe (and drawing the hormone up from the jar). Compounding pharmacies often offer pre-loaded syringes to patients for an additional fee.

And, some practitioners favor Bi-Est 2.5 mg/ml ([80:20] E3 2 mg/E2 0.5 mg) and a variety of other mixes, all of which are fine. Other carriers are commonly used that I have not recommended because there are issues with some of them. You can talk with your healthcare provider or compounding pharmacist about their preferred carriers.

There are also other novel dispensing devices, such as the "Topi-Click," various "pens," and others. They work well but are usually more expensive. In the interest of cost savings and their own excellence, the other dispensing methods listed above are just fine.

Now, I'd like to show you a few examples of *progesterone* formulations that are prepared in Carbopol and Lipoderm carriers. We'll also discuss the oral route of hormone administration. But, I'll begin by showing you common starting dosages of progesterone prepared in Carbopol.

*Perimenopause:*

- Progesterone 3% in Carbopol (common starting dosages)
  - 1 pump (15 mg, 1/2 ml) or
  - 1/8th level tsp (9 mg) or
  - 1/4 level tsp (18 mg) or
  - 1/2 or 1 ml in a syringe
  - Titration upwards can begin here

*Menopause:* when prescribing progesterone to a *menopausal* woman and/or a woman with skin absorption issues, we may want to start with a stronger concentration using similar amounts. The strongest concentration for progesterone in Carbopol is 10%. Dosages for the 10% (100 mg/ml) formulation include:

- Progesterone 10% in Carbopol
  - 1 pump = 50 mg (1.2 ml) or
  - 1/8th tsp = 60 mg or
  - 1/2 ml in a syringe = 50 mg
  - Start with 1 pump or 1/8th tsp or 0.5 ml at bedtime

At times, when absorption issues are a concern, progesterone can be formulated in Lipoderm, up to 20% (200 mg/ml):

- Progesterone 20% in Lipoderm
  - 1 pump = 100 ml
  - 1/8th level tsp = 120 mg
  - 1/2 ml in a syringe = 100 mg

*Oral Progesterone: A Common Alternative to Transdermal*

The most common alternative to transdermal progesterone is progesterone in capsules, micronized, by the oral route. This can actually be a quite common mode of treatment. Although transdermal progesterone is my initial go-to for most women, often enough, I will change to oral progesterone for the following reasons:

- At times, a patient is not absorbing sufficient progesterone by the transdermal route to balance the estrogens. A young woman's body, as previously explained, can have significantly more progesterone, milligram-for-milligram, compared to estrogens. To balance Bi-Est in treating a woman in menopause, we want a woman's body to absorb significantly more milligrams of progesterone than Bi-Est. As an example, progesterone in the organic oils is made up in 200 mg/ml concentrations, whereas a common Bi-Est formulation is 30 mg/ml.

- A patient titrates to 6 drops of transdermal progesterone and either falls shy of alleviating symptoms of insufficiency or falls shy of producing sufficient pregnanediol levels, as evidenced by 24-hour urine hormone testing. (Pregnanediol, a direct metabolite of progesterone, is used in urine hormone testing to assess progesterone levels.)

- We are seeking a special benefit for sleep than can occur from oral progesterone.

When prescribing oral progesterone, I use the following protocol:

- I most often initially prescribe two bottles of micronized progesterone, 30 capsules each: one bottle of 25 mg and one bottle 50 mg capsules. For eventual fine-tuning, at times, I'll prescribe a third bottle of 30 capsules: 5 mg each.

  ○ The starting dose is 25 mg taken before bedtime. We try this for three nights, for example.

- ○ If this is insufficient to alleviate progesterone deficiency symptoms, a woman can then titrate up to 50 mg: one 50 mg capsule.

- ○ The dosage can be increased up to 125 mg.

- ○ Common final dosages in my practice range from 50–75 mg, though some women use less or more than these dosages. I do not go above 125 mg because the pregnanediol levels, as confirmed on 24-hour urine hormone test results, exceed physiologic range.

- ○ Fine-tuning can be accomplished at any dosage level using 5 mg capsules. I have patients on less than 25 mg per night as well as on any increments of 5 mg above 25 mg.

- ○ The optimal dose is found again by titration: taking progesterone at night and waking up groggy, as if you had overdosed on a sleeping pill, is a common symptom of excess.

- ○ Some practitioners follow this regimen but begin at a 50 mg starting dose.

- The choice of regimens is based on the clinical evaluation of each individual woman, taking into account her sensitivity, for example, as well as how long her body has been without substantial progesterone.

- Again, an important additional reason for a trial of the oral route for progesterone is that it often provides a special benefit for sleep. This happens to derive from the biochemical processing of oral progesterone and is due to one of its metabolites.

Progesterone in sublingual troches:

- Progesterone can also be prepared in sublingual troches. As with all sublingual preparations, there will be mingling with saliva and the swallowing of hormones. Unlike oral estrogens and testosterone, oral progesterone is not a problem and can be fine in troches.

- Sublingual absorption can be better milligram for milligram than transdermal and oral. Lower dosages of these troches can be effective. A troche of 100 mg of progesterone can be prepared, then divided into quarters so that titration begins with a 25-milligram dose.

*Transvaginal, Translabial, and Perianal Administration: Carriers and Methods*

For administration to these areas, there are the following issues to consider:

- In general, absorption is better through the mucosal surfaces than through the skin. Therefore, lower dosages are often required.

- The carriers have to be non-astringent as these mucosal surfaces are more delicate. The organic oils are non-astringent:

  o Progesterone 200 mg/ml can be applied intravaginally, at times to great advantage if a woman is not absorbing sufficient progesterone through the skin.

  o Bi-Est 30 mg/ml 80:20 can easily be applied intra- and extra-vaginally and to the external perianal mucosa, and it can be titrated by drops.

  o Compounding pharmacists have several non-astringent carriers to offer.

- The amounts delivered need to be less in volume. These are small areas. Large quantities of a hormone/

carrier mix would be excessive. For gels and creams, the lesser volumes are created by making the concentrations stronger and administering them in 0.1 ml amounts from a 1 ml syringe.

For example:

- Bi-Est 20 mg/ml 80:20 (E3 16 mg, E2 4 mg) placed in a 1 ml syringe: each 0.1 ml delivers 0.6 mgeeq
- Bi-Est 15 mg/ml 80:20 (E3 12 mg, E2 3 mg) delivers 0.5 mgeeq/0.1 ml

*Another Commonly Used Preparation: Vaginal Estriol*

Vaginal dryness and vaginal atrophy are common problems for women in menopause. This issue is sometimes mild, sometimes moderately severe, and sometimes severe. Often, when treating a menopausal woman with Bi-Est, over time, the vagina will restore to a reasonably healthy or healthy state as she titrates her transdermally applied hormones to symptom-relieving dosages. This can take one to six months, depending on several factors.

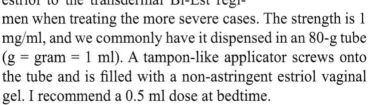

At times, we add a tube of vaginal estriol to the transdermal Bi-Est regimen when treating the more severe cases. The strength is 1 mg/ml, and we commonly have it dispensed in an 80-g tube (g = gram = 1 ml). A tampon-like applicator screws onto the tube and is filled with a non-astringent estriol vaginal gel. I recommend a 0.5 ml dose at bedtime.

While lying down, you would insert the vaginal applicator as high up into the vagina as it will easily go and dispense 0.5 ml of estriol (the syringe is marked). If you continue to lay down, the gel will better remain in the vagina. By the time one tube is used (160 days!), there is rarely need to prescribe a second tube as the general body levels of Bi-Est (which has been applied to the forearms, for example) should be sufficient to support the ongoing health of the vagina.

In addition, at times, testosterone and/or DHEA will be added to the vaginal estriol prescription as each, or both together can support vaginal recovery.

One most important reason to support the health of the vagina is because it is supportive to the health of the bladder. The urethra, the opening of the tube that comes from the bladder, ends in the vagina. When the vaginal mucosa contiguous to the urethra is healthier, urethral irritation from an atrophic vagina can heal. When the vagina is atrophic, that opening (the urethral meatus) is easily irritated and vulnerable to recurrent bladder infections. This can provoke urinary urgency, even incontinence, of small amounts or large. This, along with the loss of bladder support from depleted androgens and no exercise of the bladder/vagina/rectum support muscle (the levator ani), ultimately, can result in the need for adult diapers/underpants.

This does not exhaust the description of the number of carriers or the number of dispensing methods. But, it should provide sufficient background for you to understand almost any bio-identical hormones your health professional prescribes for you.

*A Final Note About Dosages and Testing*

No matter what transdermal hormone preparation you use—organic oils, gels, or creams—and no matter what dosage, strength and ratio (for Bi-Est), the most important thing I want you to remember is that once you have stabilized on your regimen, it is imperative that you do the 24-hour urine hormone test. Because women vary so much in their ability to absorb any hormone that is applied to the skin, what matters most is what is absorbed into the body. I find that only the 24-hour urine hormone test can accurately detect this. I have treated women with doses of Bi-Est high enough that I was concerned about the outcomes only to see that their estrogen levels were in the optimal range, or even below. Vice versa, I have also treated women with doses that I thought would be too low to help them, and the test results showed that their estrogen was in the optimal range!

*Initial Use of Androgens?*

There is a possibility that the androgens will be prescribed at consistent small dosages at the beginning of treatment—most often in the case of obvious significant testosterone and DHEA deficiencies. Many women will not start with these hormones as more often than not they usually do not have an androgen deficiency at the beginning of menopause. I find it best to keep the number of initial hormones to two (Bi-Est and progesterone) so that a woman can best get a sense of each of these hormones. Sooner or later, the androgens (testosterone and DHEA) will diminish. Once this occurs, it is very important to replenish them.

Chapter Eleven

# Androgens

Androgens are a family of hormones, the two most important of which are testosterone and DHEA. Testosterone? For women? So many of you have already heard that testosterone is a very important hormone for women. Although women do not have as much testosterone as men, it is essential for muscle mass and strength. Stamina, libido, orgasm, mood, and energy also depend on its presence.

Figure 11a below lists the symptoms of testosterone deficiency. These include diminished libido, energy and stamina, sense of security, hair loss, flabbiness (especially of the upper arms and cheeks), and muscular weakness. Weak muscles, with loss of muscle mass, known to doctors as sarcopenia, can lead to difficulty in rising from a chair and, ultimately, to instability in standing and walking. In medical school, this was emphasized to me by a gerontologist (a specialist in treating the elderly). As I mentioned before, I so clearly remember this doctor telling us that one

**Finding Your Optimal Dose**                    Figure 11a.

TESTOSTERONE

Too little:
- Diminished libido*
- Loss of sense of security
- Body hair loss
- Diminished energy/stamina
- Flabbiness/muscular weakness
  (upper arms, thighs, & cheeks)

Too much:
- Hyper-aggressiveness
- Excessive oiliness of skin
- Increased pimples/acne
- Increased hair growth
  on body, face, &/or
  place of application

The Menopause Method

of the main medical issues plaguing older adults is sarcopenia, as it leads to stance and gait instability and falling. Too often those falls are onto weak bones, thus, fracturing hips, etc.

Weakness can include the pelvic floor muscles that support the bladder. This weakness, coupled with vaginal atrophy, with its accompanying irritation to the urethra (the tube leading from the bladder to the vagina) can lead to bladder issues galore. As a result, a woman can develop urinary frequency, urgency, frequent urination at night, losing urine on a cough, and urinary incontinence — all from losing this crucial bladder support and urethral irritation. Elderly women often turn to "Depends." I can tell you that many of them do not like these adult diapers and are embarrassed by them, as necessary as they can become. Replenishing androgens and exercising, including the pelvic floor muscle, along with restoring vaginal health: an ounce of prevention can be worth a ton of cure.

Testosterone is produced in the ovaries and the adrenal glands. As estrogen and progesterone production from the ovaries declines, then stops entirely, testosterone continues to be produced in the ovaries (at least for a while) as well as in the adrenal glands. For this reason, some women enter perimenopause and early menopause with adequate or substantial levels of testosterone. These women will not require testosterone treatment initially. "Initially?" Alas, sooner or later, testosterone output from the ovaries diminishes. Depending on stress levels, even adrenal testosterone can decline. The upshot is that sooner or later in menopause (usually between two to five years), women develop low testosterone levels and are affected by it. As an aside, estrogens are produced primarily in the ovaries;

when ovarian estrogen production ceases, most estrogen is gone. Interestingly, testosterone can be converted into estradiol in the fat cells. As a result, heavier set women will have more estradiol produced from this conversion. This is not nearly enough, however, to form an endometrial lining and menstruate. Yet, there can be a sufficient amount to stave off estrogen inadequacy symptoms. It is common to see thinner menopausal women have more hot flashes and other symptoms. Many heavier set women do not have these symptoms and wonder, what is the "big deal" about menopause? Thinner women may have to face more hormonal deficiency symptoms; however, they are spared the consequences of the excessive weight.

There can be a bit more to achieving correct testosterone levels. As I mentioned, progesterone and estrogen loss is great by the onset of menopause, but the diminishing of testosterone is variable. For some women, testosterone even increases during perimenopause and early menopause. At times, this will cause increased facial hair or acne. Other perimenopausal or early menopausal women will have pronounced androgen deficiency symptoms. In these women, low testosterone was caused by longstanding stress that depleted the androgens.

Most commonly, we begin treatment with Bi-Est and progesterone alone in women who have adequate androgens. Lack of androgen deficiency symptoms are the clue to the status of these women. In women with no obvious initial androgen needs, it is convenient to bypass, at least initially, treatment with both testosterone and DHEA. It gives these women months to a few years to become proficient at achieving sufficient estrogen and progesterone levels and balance before bringing in additional hormonal treatment variables. Conversely, when women have obvious androgen deficiency at the outset of perimenopause or menopause, we do begin testosterone and DHEA treatment along with the Bi-Est and progesterone.

As with other hormones, the amount of testosterone you need depends upon what your body has been accustomed to and how much production you have lost. Before treating with testosterone (except for those women with obvious symptoms), I prefer to test. Ultimately, as with other hormones, confirmatory testing to assure safe levels is very important. The most common approach to hormone treatment begins with Bi-Est and progesterone. This allows women to take the time they need, usually months, to alleviate symptoms and arrive at what they feel are optimal dosages. At that time, I test their hormone levels (see the next chapter on hormone testing). From that testing, I will get an accurate assessment of the androgen levels and choose to add testosterone and DHEA treatment—or not—depending on the test results.

*Treatment with Testosterone*

Dose titration of testosterone follows the same protocol as other hormones:

- Start with a lowish dose.

- Titrate up to an optimal dose based on the symptoms of deficiency and excess as summarized in Figure 11a. Excess testosterone leads to excessive aggressiveness, an excessive oiliness of the skin, acne, and hair growth where it is applied. Additionally, hair growth can appear on the face.

- You may have to adjust progesterone and/or estrogen dosages once you introduce testosterone. This is due

---

**Finding Your Optimal Dose**                                    Figure 11a.

TESTOSTERONE

Too little:
- Diminished libido*
- Loss of sense of security
- Body hair loss
- Diminished energy/stamina
- Flabbiness/muscular weakness
  (upper arms, thighs, & cheeks)

Too much:
- Hyper-aggressiveness
- Excessive oiliness of skin
- Increased pimples/acne
- Increased hair growth
  on body, face, &/or
  place of application

 Menopause Method

---

to all of the biochemical interrelationships occurring between these hormones.

For testosterone, I also recommend the organic oils preparation. Most often, I begin with a 5 mg/ml dosage:

- Apply 1 or 2 drops to the external perianal mucosa.

- Testosterone can also be applied to the area of the clitoris, the outside of the inner vaginal lips, the perineum (the space between the vagina and the anus), or the pubic hair region.

- If a woman is not having intercourse, it can be applied in the vagina.

- You can apply it to many regions of the body. However, if you apply it to an area that has hair follicles, you are likely to enhance hair growth in that area.

- Because testosterone can convert to estradiol, I suggest you do not apply it to the areas where estrogen application is not appropriate.

- Apply it once daily in the morning or 1/2 hour before intercourse. (It has been known to enhance orgasm!)

- Another common dosage that can be used: 10 mg/ml.

---

Figure 11b.

## Testosterone Hormone Application

- Usually in the morning, although an optional time can be 1/2 hour before intercourse (as it may enhance orgasm).
- Apply it to the external perianal mucosa area, the clitoral area, the pubic hair region, around the vagina, and the perineum (the space between the vagina and anus). Caution: give it time to absorb into these regions, or your partner could absorb the extra hormone.
- Testosterone is also available in a non-hydroalcoholic skin gel, which is preferred if you are going to use a gel on mucosal areas.
- Estriol &/or testosterone vaginal gels are available if indicated (available in a non-hydroalcoholic gel), and both can be excellent in assisting the return of vaginal health.

---

Another preparation is Carbopol, which is a hydro-alcoholic gel:

- 4 mg/2.5 ml (1.6 mg/g)

- Begin with 0.3 cc or 1/16th teaspoon

- For some vaginal conditions, such as a more severe atrophic form of vaginitis, testosterone in the organic oils or a special non-alcoholic preparation can be used and combined with estriol for application in the vagina.

*Treatment with DHEA*

As I mentioned earlier, sooner or later the androgens will decline. In menopausal women, DHEA is produced in the adrenal glands. A woman can enter menopause with a variable amount of DHEA production. Some women in their forties and fifties maintain a sufficient output of DHEA; however, it is unusual to see levels as high as those in younger women. More often than not, women begin to have significant androgen deficiency during perimenopause. I believe it

---

is because the androgens can serve the additional function of providing "firepower" for the biological stress response: excessive responses to stress eventually leads to low levels of DHEA.

Although DHEA is the most prevalent of the steroid hormones, it does not exhibit clear-cut, obvious symptoms of decline as do the estrogens, progesterone, and testosterone. You will not find DHEA listed on any of our charts that show the symptoms of hormone insufficiency. No worries — testing reveals all. Prior to any treatment, a routine blood test requesting the "DHEA-S" level will help determine the status of this hormone. It is important that your practitioner order the DHEA-Sulfate ("DHEA-S") form when measuring blood levels of DHEA to obtain a proper assessment. And, as always, a 24-hour urine test reveals the full androgen picture. This test also shows the androgen metabolites (androsterone and etiocholanolone are the principal ones), which can be very helpful in assessing the androgen levels.

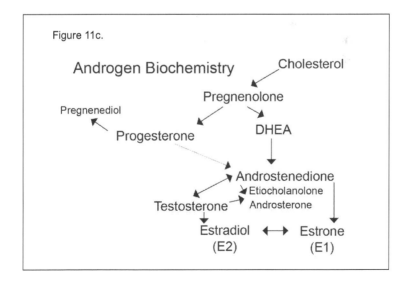

Figure 11c.

Androgen Biochemistry

DHEA treatment can be transdermal or oral. To say it once again, it does not rise to the highest bar of health and safety to administer estrogens or testosterone by mouth. And, as I have mentioned, progesterone is not only fine by the oral route, at times it is referred.

- Transdermally, my "go-to" Rx for DHEA is 100 mg/ml in the organic oils, applied to the pubic hair region or perineum once daily (usually in the morning). One drop contains 4 mg of DHEA.

- Because DHEA is safe in the oral form, quite often I'll prescribe it in a compounded capsule. Many patients appreciate the convenience of supplementing orally with DHEA. Because it is fat soluble, it is best to take it with breakfast or another meal.

- Most of my patients do very well on either 10 or 15 mg. Some even need less than 10 mg. The optimal amount is ultimately determined by 24-hour urine assessment of DHEA, testosterone, and their metabolites. Again, unlike estrogens, progesterone, and testosterone, there are no easy clinical signs or symptoms of DHEA insufficiency or excess. (Thus, you do not see DHEA listed on the Symptoms Chart.)

- It should not be necessary to treat a woman with more than 15 mg per day of oral DHEA. It is of concern to many of us that DHEA is so readily available "over-the-counter" in oral forms and at higher, 25 mg dosages. 24-hour urine hormone test results will invariably reveal excessive amounts of DHEA if > 15 mg are taken orally. Some women will even show excessive amounts of DHEA in the urine test on 15 mg.

- Reading between the lines: 24-hour urine hormone testing is so important for yet another reason!

# Chapter Twelve

# Additional Details About Hormone Treatment

*Important Variations and Alternatives with Hormones*

In the preceding chapters, I have suggested many basic guidelines about hormone treatment. However, many individual variations and exceptions are possible such as these:

- Some women need or prefer to apply progesterone twice daily.

- To better alleviate nighttime hot flashes and sleep disturbance, certain women apply additional estrogen at bedtime.

- There are also women who become too energized from estrogen and have difficulty sleeping if they apply estrogens too late in the evening. So, they will often apply their second dose of estrogen late in the afternoon.

- In some cases, progesterone does not absorb well through the skin, and the oral or sublingual form is necessary.

- Although uncommon, some women do not feel well on any estrogen.

- There are some instances where excessive progesterone will lead to estrogen deficiency symptoms. Because progesterone also binds to estrogen receptor sites, although far less avidly than estrogen binds, excessive progesterone by the "law of chemical mass action" can displace estrogen from its receptor sites and lead to estrogen deficiency symptoms.

- Excessive progesterone dosage can result in estrogen dominance symptoms, as we mention on the "Finding Your Optimal Dose" symptom chart as the "unusual progesterone effect."

- There is the rare situation where a woman feels uncomfortable on almost any dose of progesterone. Often, these women had early total hysterectomies and were not treated with hormones or were treated with estrogens only. As a result, their progesterone receptor sites have gone dormant, and even a little bit of progesterone can feel like a flood. Sometimes, this can be remedied by beginning with minuscule dosages of progesterone and gradually increasing the dosages over time.

- Although rare, if you have developed thrombophlebitis or even achy lower extremities or achy veins while on the birth control pill, you should be especially cautious about using progesterone or should avoid using it at all.

- There can be other idiosyncrasies in hormone treatment. This underlines the importance for you to find a properly trained, skilled, and experienced physician or nurse practitioner to assist you!

*Other Variables*

We can develop good plans for your hormone therapy but, ultimately, the "proof is in the pudding." If a woman is on a treatment program and does not feel right, something definitely is not right! Conversely, when a woman begins to feel better, we are usually close to or have reached an optimal hormone treatment program. However, ultimately, "feeling better" must be confirmed with proper testing. It is essential that we use safe doses (not excessive doses), that estrogens are being biochemically processed (metabolized) correctly, and that a sufficient amount of progesterone is absorbed, etc.

Throughout history, millions, perhaps billions, of women have *not* received menopausal hormone treatment. That is not inferring they all did well. Many did not! Yet, many did fine. There are also many women who prefer not to supplement with hormones and can still achieve satisfying results from a proper diet, nutritional supplements and, at times, herbal products. Many good practitioners have other methods they prefer. In contrast, many women do not succeed with these non-hormonal approaches alone. The increased risks that occur from low hormone levels in women who are not receiving hormone treatment, once again, need to be cosidered.

The possible use of herbs for the treatment of menopause raises another question. Herbs contain molecules that are non-identical to those in our body; thus, technically, they are "medicines." The body integrates identical molecules (such as foods), yet reacts to the non-identical. It is this reaction to non-identical molecules that we capitalize on for medicinal effect. Use of any medicine, including herbs, is best prescribed for a given period of time and, ideally, should not be used long-term. Therefore, herbs, in my opinion, may not be ideally suited for long-term treatment.

So, what is the best approach for you? Once again, it will all come down to your individual situation regarding all of your medical details, risks, preferences, intuition, and knowing. It will be your personal wise choice!

*If Hormones Are Right, They Feel Right*

If hormones are right for you, they are going to feel right, and you will have a sense of well-being. This is important! People who need hormones and take the right ones in the right doses feel better! If you do not feel well from taking hormones, something is wrong, and changes need to be made. In this case, professional assistance is often necessary.

There are, however, exceptions to what I have just stated! Some women who are supplementing with hormones feel as if things are fine, or even "great," yet when we evaluate their hormone levels by 24-hour urine hormone testing, they are not fine! This situation is not common, but it does occur. Examples include:

- The hormone levels are elevated, but there are no symptoms or signs of excess. At times, a woman will titrate up to and above optimal hormone levels into excessive levels. This will be revealed by 24-hour testing. In the long run, this elevation is not beneficial in my opinion. A small percentage of women feel "good" or "great" on excessive hormone levels. The template for this relates to the high hormone levels that are present during pregnancy: some women feel terrific with these high levels, yet many do not. Our medical, scientific studies very much call into question the safety of high levels of hormones during menopause.[12.1]

- The estrogens are not elevated. However, they are not biochemically processing in a preferred and safe way.

- The ovarian hormone dosages or body levels are not typical. For example, the dosages appear more robust than is common (it will take the knowledge and experience of your professional provider to be aware of this). It will appear as if the hormones are not functioning properly: dosages are ample or robust but symptoms are not being relieved. This problem can stem from elevations in sex hormone binding globulin (SHBG), a transport protein, that can pose a significant challenge to dosage determination.

  Elevated levels of SHBG can result from earlier birth control pill usage as well as higher-than-optimal dosages of estrogen, testosterone, and even thyroid hormone. This issue is a subject for your medical professional! Because excessive levels of SHBG are not that uncommon and will consequently cause the excessive binding of hormones, I always order a SHBG serum level along with initial routine blood tests. Having that baseline level can be very helpful.

A hormone to "watch" is estrogen. At times, a woman can experience dramatic relief when she begins estrogen therapy. Over time, the initial doses used may turn out to be excessive, and symptoms of too much estrogen can sneak up on you. Although the majority of women who "slip" into high dosages of estrogen do feel it and experience the symptoms of excess, overdose is not always clear cut. I have consulted with women who do not feel well from excess estrogen but do not necessarily develop a classic overdose symptom, such as breast tenderness. I have also experienced situations where the initial treatment with estrogen led to the successful alleviation of deficiency symptoms, but with continued use, some patients regressed, and their symptoms reoccurred. It can appear as if the estrogens are not working or absorbing. So, it seemed as if the next step would be to increase the estrogen, yet this only led to continued deficiency symptoms and diminished well-being. Testing revealed estrogen excess! Once again, the explanation for continued deficiency symptoms may involve elevations of SHBG. Testing is not difficult or expensive. To me, "testing is queen."

Ah, yes. Though the vast majority of hormonal treatment programs develop and proceed smoothly, there are some that require extra effort and diligence. And there are a few that require a medical professional with the utmost in experience and/or issue-solving skills, along with your patience during the discovery process. I think this might be why "patients" are so called: you are all so often called upon to be patient!

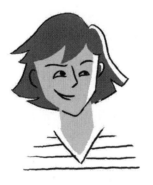

I'm not stressed by
menopause, are you?

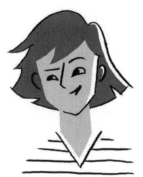

Menopause,
Schemopause!

Chapter Thirteen

# Treating Elderly Women with Hormones

*A View From Several Perspectives*

Ever since the Women's Health Initiative (WHI) study brought the concern of hormones to the public and medical professionals, there has been a reticence, even fear, of hormones. At the time of this writing, there are policy recommendations of general medical consensus to avoid treating women in menopause with hormones for an extended period, perhaps, no more than five to ten years. In Chapter Three, I have examined the risks and benefits of hormone therapy. In our professional training program, The Menopause Method, I explore this subject in considerable depth.

Treating elderly women with hormones raises the risk/benefit issue. The complete picture is not entirely clear! Risks exist, for sure. In general, the risk of a wide variety of serious illnesses and death definitely abound for the elderly! Specifically, as it relates to hormones, if a woman is harboring a small estrogen receptor-site-positive cancer, that cancer would very likely have its growth facilitated by estrogen therapy. In contrast, if an elderly woman were to remain at an almost-zero estrogen level, which is common for her age demographic, the cancer might remain extremely slow-growing.

The risk for breast cancer, independent of hormone treatment, exists. The disease process of cancer is quite complex. So many factors can play into its development —

or not. An assessment of specific risks, in this case for breast cancer, is important in the evaluation of treating an elderly woman or any woman with hormones.

Another concern when treating the elderly with hormones, specifically estrogen, relates to arteriosclerosis and blood clotting. We know for certain that there is an increasingly high prevalence of arteriosclerosis as a woman ages. The roughened surface of an artery injured by arteriosclerosis is more vulnerable to become the very area that provokes the formation of a blood clot. These clots are so often the cause of heart attacks and strokes. A finding in the WHI study showed a small but definite increase in strokes and heart attacks in women treated with the *combined* estrogen/progestin, Prempro. This is an important aspect of widespread concern, especially for the elderly. The most crucial issue here is that the "combined equine estrogen/progestin" *does* increase the propensity for blood to clot. Knowledge of this is widespread in the medical world as well as the general public. However, the problem of increased blood coagulability with oral estrogens is not as well-known.[13.1] Quite the opposite has been found for *transdermal* estrogens: they *reduce* the propensity for blood coagulation![13.1]

On the other hand, there are plenty of risks associated with the dramatically low levels of estrogens, progesterone, and androgens, which are a certainty in all women as they advance in age and, often, in those who are much younger.[13.2] Most often, the common garden variety and disdained challenges of the elderly are often directly related to hormonal insufficiency. I have spoken at length in previous chapters of the cognitive decline, arteriosclerosis, stance and gait instability, muscle loss and weakness, bladder issues (from vaginal atrophy and urethral irritation coupling with bladder muscle support weakness), and a propensity to fall onto osteoporotic bones, etc., etc., etc. At times, elderly women are willing to admit to these very challenging issues, and if you do not realize this already, they are often very disturbed by them. I am certain that those of you who are elderly, or those of you caring for your elderly mother, are acutely aware of what I am talking about.

In other words, as I teach in our live and online training programs for physicians and nurse practitioners, "there may be risks associated with the hormonal treatment of the elderly; however, there are a near certainty of difficulties from no treatment."

> ***There may be risks associated with the hormonal treatment of the elderly; however, there are a near certainty of difficulties from no treatment.***

*Medicine Up Close and Personal*

I was launched into this subject by some of the health issues that arose in my mother and mother-in-law. First, was the onset of significant cognitive decline of my mother in her late eighties, sufficient to be of major concern to my father and our family. I began treating her with hormones. Before that time, she had never used them. Like so many women of her generation, she saw no reason to, never did, and had no interest. However, she did accede to my father and my wishes, and, to our delight, within six months, she had returned to 80% function! I happened to test her before treatment, and you can see her values in Appendix A. After a few years, she discontinued treatment on her own. Three years later, in her early nineties, she began needing a walker and cane because of lower extremity weakness. We resumed hormonal treatment, and within three months, she had retired her walker and cane. Hormonal treatment gave her a year or two more with decent function, although, ultimately, cognition and the ability to walk declined.

My mother-in-law was also in her late eighties. She had a total hysterectomy in her thirties with no hormonal treatment. By the time she was in her fifties, stents were inserted, followed by coronary bypass surgery in her sixties. By her eighties, she had suffered her third heart attack. She was extremely weak in her lower extremities, so weak that she could not get out of a chair on her own. This weakness led to her losing her balance in the kitchen, falling to the floor, fracturing her osteoporotic pelvis and humerus. You can view her hormone test results in Appendix A as well. Six months after starting her on hormone replenishing, she was able to walk and get up out of a chair without even needing to use her arms. You can see a video of her and my mother on our professional website, www.menopausemethod.com. From the home page, select "For Medical Professionals"; then, click on MM-Elder.

From these origins, we developed a hormone formulation for elderly women. It is available in both the organic oils base as well as a Carbopol-plus base. The formulation contains Bi-Est, progesterone, testosterone, DHEA, and pregnenolone. With all that I have explained about

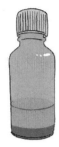 the advantages of the organic oils as well as the need to address menopausal treatment with individual hormones, MM-Elder for Women is different! I can tell you that in this case, it is necessary to blend all of the hormones into one bottle. Few elderly women can easily comply with several individual hormone bottles.

Also, when we assess that it is unlikely that a given patient will remember or be able to shake the oils mixture version of MM-Elder, we prescribe the Carbopol version. Carbopol is a solvent capable of dissolving all of the hormones. This formulation does not require shaking and primarily calls for one pump application per day to the soft forearm. It has to be this simple for many of the elderly (trust me), and that is why we made this version available.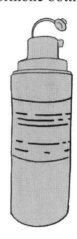

MM-Elder is available in two different strengths. One is the standard version, MM-Elder, which is the one I used on my mother. We also have a half-strength version, MM-Elder-S, for more sensitive patients. For a few reasons, there are some women that we prefer to start on the half-strength formulation. Then, provided they tolerate that well (without symptoms of hormonal excess), after one month of starting treatment, they could increase the MM-Elder-S formulation up to two pumps per day. We have had one elderly patient on MM-Elder for Women develop breast tenderness. Hence, the creation of a half-strength version, -S. I had no hesitation prescribing the standard strength for my mother, and she tolerated it very well. Some physicians and nurse practitioners may want to start with the "-S" formulation on their specific patient for understandable reasons.

We do not have the intention of prolonging the inevitable leaving of our beloved planet. Nor is MM-Elder capable of doing this: the benefits of hormones lasted only for so long for both my beloved mother-in-law and mother. However, it is our intention to help make our precious elders' remaining time on Earth as healthy and as functional as possible.

Chapter Fourteen

# Patient Assessment: Initial and Ongoing

The key to developing the most successful and safest menopause treatment program begins with learning about the health details of the patient. Assessment begins with the medical history. As I mentioned in Chapter Five, as part of The Menopause Method, an extensive questionnaire is available to all new patients of any Menopause Method trained practitioner. Before the first consultation, the questionnaire is completed online and will automatically transmit securely to the practitioner.

At the time of the first consultation, the questionnaire is reviewed, and the following process occurs:

- If the consultation is conducted in-person in the physician's or nurse practitioner's office, a physical examination will be performed. If not in-person, thus via telemedicine, the woman's personal gynecologist or health care provider will be doing the complete physical and female exam.

- All relevant and recent medical reports will be reviewed, such as blood tests, mammograms, bone density test results, etc.

During the first visit, so much is learned about the patient. Unless an unexpected medical priority emerges, it is customary to prescribe the initial hormone program, as described in the previous chapters.

A perimenopausal or menopausal woman will have a list of symptoms that suggest ovarian hormone insufficiency.

Various forms of biochemical tests are available to define another view of hormonal levels beyond these subjective symptoms. There are also numerous fundamental methods to assess basic female health that are relevant and important, some of which are enumerated in Figure 14a.

Figure 14a.  Patient Assessment

Initial Evaluation:
  Medical history: review initial questionnaire
  Office physical examination (unless by telemedicine)
  Review of recent and previous test results

Possible Initial Testing (optional, based upon need):
  Blood tests, breast and pelvic exams
  (with pap smear), hormone testing, mammogram,
  thermogram, and bone density

Hormone Testing:
  At the time an optimal hormone program is achieved
  (usually 3 to 6 months), or whenever more information
  is needed during the dose discovery process

Periodic Testing:
  Annual follow-up questionnaire
  Annual female exam, blood testing, 24-hour urine
  hormone testing, mammogram, thermogram,
  bone density, and transvaginal ultrasound (time
  between each test varies with the individual patient)

*Hormonal Testing: Introduction*

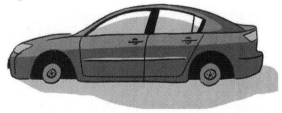

Hormone testing is valuable, interesting, and always *crucial* to an ongoing successful treatment program. A pinnacle moment in seminars I present to physicians, nurse practitioners, and prescribing compounding pharmacists occurs when I display the PowerPoint slide of a car with no wheels onto the screen, saying "To drive a car, we must

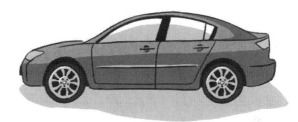

have wheels; to treat women in menopause, we must do the 24-hour urine hormone test." I pause, then repeat that sentence. I pause again. I wait until I see that this statement has settled in a bit... then I go on to elaborate. It's a bit of a shocker. We were not taught about this test in our early professional training. It's a learning curve to understand and interpret it, which is why there is often a mental "gasp" in the audience (see the examples of 24-hour urine hormone test results in Appendix A).

24-hour urine hormone testing is absolutely indispensable for safety and accuracy of treatment. I am emphatic about this, though some professionals will challenge this assertion.

To make the treatment of women in menopause as safe as we possibly can, one of the benchmarks is precision dosing of hormones: *not too little and not too much*. There is *only* one single method that I know of that is capable of doing precisely that, and that is the 24-hour urine hormone test. The parameters of optimal ranges we have developed are surmised from critical sources: our medical literature, and known testing norms. The scientific studies (see many of them relevant to safety in Appendix B), when carefully evaluated, provide great information to define optimal ranges and safe limits!

And, sorry to say, it is too easy to be fooled by trying to rely on a patient's symptoms and/or the amount of dosage prescribed. For example:

- *Symptoms.* The "titration" dose determination method of starting on a low dose and gradually increasing until symptoms of hormonal insufficiency are alleviated (up to and then backing down from symptoms of excess) is a wonderful tool. If a woman has started on a low-ish dose of Bi-Est and gradually increases the dosage, alleviating symptoms, but then as she increases, begins to feel breast tenderness, we know that she has titrated to excess—a safety bumper. I cannot begin to count the number of women in my practice alone that have been so served and delighted by this method. It works so well... *most but not all of the time!* There are a certain number of women who will increase their dose above the common norms without experiencing overdose symptoms. I have explained this to myself by remembering the days I delivered babies and the many women who felt quite buoyed up by the much-increased estrogen and progesterone levels of pregnancy: enlarging and tender breasts were easily understood, not as improper or hormonal overdose, but as the ultimate preparation for breastfeeding. The moral of this story: though not most common, but often enough, a woman can titrate above what is needed, feel good, and have a

24-hour urine hormone test result that reveals excessive and even greatly elevated amounts of estrogens.

- *Dosage amounts and potency.* If we evaluated the final amount of Bi-Est dosage a patient was using after titration, and the actual number seemed too low or even too high, we simply could not rely on dosage potency and amount alone. There is such a remarkable variation of absorption through the skin, one woman to the next. This variability is dependent upon qualities such as the health and relative youthfulness of the skin. Thus, a woman could be applying what seems at first look to the medical provider as a very high dose—which we would want to avoid—and lower. However, 24-hour urine hormone testing could reveal normal range estrogens, or even below normal, if the woman's skin was not absorbing well. Vice versa: if the medical provider learned from their patient the Bi-Est dose was quite low, by comparative norms, it would still be possible for test results to show normal or even elevated estrogen levels. This could occur if the patient's skin, in this case, was very healthy and youthful and thus had exuberant absorption of the transdermal hormones!

- *Other hormone testing methods.* Blood and saliva tests, to me, are simply not reliable for reasons of time-from-preceding dose, and other issues, to detect with the clarity and precision that 24-hour urine hormone testing does.

In our Menopause Method training program, we are highly specific as to what values we consider to be optimal for the amounts of each of the hormones. From stem to stern, in bottle design, amounts provided in the bottles, optimal drop suggestions ("2 & 3" for Bi-Est), there are built-in protections against an overdose! Our newest iteration of The Menopause Method calculates the number of drops needed per month quite precisely. Thus, if a woman runs out of her hormones before a month has elapsed, she might call her prescriber or the pharmacist and ask, "Why is it that I did not have enough hormones to last a full month?" And the answer will be: "It is most likely that you titrated up to dosage levels higher than what were carefully designed and described to you."

And, no matter how much we have evolved our methods and how much care we have put into preventing an overdose, 20% of my patients, for one reason or another, when tested, will reveal dosages that I would not want to sustain over the long haul. This is why we insist upon 24-hour urine hormone testing, usually occurring at the time a woman has determined her optimal dose by titration and how she feels, and then every one to two years thereafter!

The lesson to be learned here: embrace the 24-hour urine hormone test. You will learn to appreciate it so deeply. At the time of this writing, it can still be obtained for a little less or a little more than $300. To me, it is by far one of the best bargains in laboratory medicine.

## *Hormonal Testing: Some Delightful Details*

You may have been surprised when I mentioned in Chapter Five that I very rarely test hormone levels in a new perimenopausal or menopausal patient. Once again, during perimenopause, hormone levels are variable day-to-day, often with levels erratically spiking and dipping deep (Figure 14b, next page, middle graph). Because of this, misleading information is encountered when testing. For example, a perimenopausal woman could be experiencing night sweats

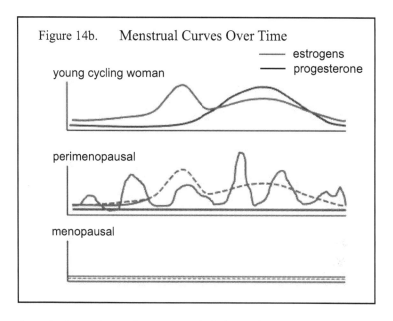

Figure 14b.     Menstrual Curves Over Time

—— estrogens
—— progesterone

young cycling woman

perimenopausal

menopausal

(an obvious sign of estrogen deficiency). But, if you test her on a day when her estrogen levels are spiking high (because the pituitary gland is trying to revive a flagging ovary), you could be misled to believe that she did not require estrogen treatment. Consider, also, that for a woman in early menopause, who has symptoms of estrogen deficiency, it would be unwise to spend her money on testing hormone levels. Only what is already so obvious will be learned: that her estrogen and progesterone levels are very low. Early in my career, I learned this by testing many women in early menopause. The classic symptoms were all there: absence of periods, hot flashes, memory issues, etc. Sophisticated 24-hour urine hormone testing revealed very low estrogens and progesterone levels. No surprise! It didn't take too long for me to realize that there was no value in testing perimenopausal or early menopausal women.

There are a few exceptions. If a new patient is uncomfortable initiating hormone therapy without having her hormone levels tested (even after my explanations), and she has the financial resources, fine, I am happy to order testing. A second exception occurs when the medical history gives me concern that there may be more going on hormonally than just low ovarian output, for example, low adrenal corticosteroid production. I will also order initial hormone testing on these women.

Regardless of our initial choice to test or not, our approach in The Menopause Method is that every female patient's hormone levels are always tested at the right time. Preferably, that "right time" occurs when symptoms have been alleviated, and hormone treatment dosages are stabilized. Most commonly, this takes place two to four months after initiating treatment. We also test hormone levels every one to two years after that. Once dosages have stabilized, we test levels to learn the following:

- Are the hormone levels within what I consider to be the optimal range? Not too high and not too low.

- Is progesterone absorbing sufficiently?

- Are estrogens processing (metabolizing) in an optimal way?

- Are the androgen and corticosteroid levels optimal? If androgen therapy is not currently prescribed, would there be a benefit at this time?

There can be reasons to test *prior* to arriving at optimal clinical hormone levels:

- When initial attempts at treatment do not succeed, further assessment is necessary. At times, a woman can titrate to excessive dosages, and symptoms of insufficiency occur because the excessive levels of hormones interfere with proper hormone function. The clinical picture may be unclear enough that we need to test for clarification.

• When there are significant risk factors for breast, uterine, or ovarian issues, testing can be imperative early on.

One phenomenal advantage with bio-identical hormones is that medical laboratory testing can reveal the hormone levels present in a woman receiving treatment. This ability to accurately assess hormone levels while a woman is taking her hormones is special and unique to the 24-hour urine hormone testing method. This was not the case for women treated with the horse estrogens found in Premarin (half of which are not present in the female body), as they were not testable by common laboratory methods. Testing was not possible with the artificial progestins, such as Provera, Prempro, medroxyprogesterone acetate, and the progestins found in birth control pills. The progestins were problematic in their own right, beyond being non-testable!

As for the method of testing, you may have already guessed that I certainly have my favorite: hormone testing on a 24-hour collection of urine. This test has unique features:

• We receive a real-time assessment of the hormone dosage levels that a patient is taking, as the urine collection is occurring while the patient is using the hormones.

• With a 24-hour urine collection, there is no time-sampling error (Figure 14c on the following page): we receive an accurate and complete picture of how much of the hormone dosage is being absorbed in 24 hours. This information provides essential insight for your physician or nurse practitioner.

- This test assesses the hormone metabolites which I find to be crucial for understanding dosages. The metabolites are not tested or reported in blood or saliva testing. Metabolites are also related to risk: improper metabolization can confer risk.

- In my opinion, 24-hour urine hormone testing is the best financial bargain in the world of medical testing. The test ranges from $156 to $325 (current prices at the time of this publication), and at times, it is covered by insurance.

Serum and saliva testing are *time dependent:* because single samples are collected, the time following the previous dose is crucial. You will see far different hormone levels one hour after administering the previous hormone dose compared to 4 hours, 8 hours, or 24 hours afterward just because of the way hormones are absorbed (Figure 14c).

For the reasons given, I am not an advocate of blood or saliva hormone testing in perimenopausal or menopaus-

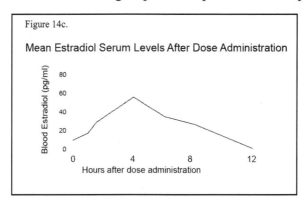

Figure 14c.

Mean Estradiol Serum Levels After Dose Administration

al women. There certainly is a place for blood testing in regularly menstruating young women. For completeness, testing must be done three-quarters of the way through a monthly cycle (for example, on day 20 of a 28-day cycle). If a young woman has irregular cycles, testing of any kind can be confusing as hormone levels are so dependent upon where a woman is in her cycle. (See the upcoming section: "Time to Test.") Salivary testing, with saliva collections taken approximately every three days, does have some use as a less expensive way to test for ovulation in young women. Saliva can also be helpful for testing the timing of cortisol and DHEA secretion in a 24-hour period.

Having given you my preference and opinions, most practitioners have their preferred methods of testing and their favorite laboratories. By observing results from a specific testing method and a specific lab, a practitioner will learn a great deal about hormones and will experience how lab results correlate with individual patients and their symptoms. This level of practical experience over a significant amount of time is crucial. In understanding and interpreting laboratory tests, nothing will replace the personal experience of an individual health practitioner using reasonable methods and good laboratories in the long-term process of testing and correlating lab results with many of their patients.

*Hormonal Testing: Reference Ranges*

One of the key pitfalls in hormonal testing or, for that matter, biochemical testing of any kind, is the issue of "normal ranges." Limitations derive from how "normal" is defined. In actual practice, no matter what the test, a given laboratory will look at a certain number of test results of any given analyte and will define normal by mathematical, statistical methods. For example, a laboratory will select the results from thousands of consecutive patients who had their blood drawn for fasting glucose determination. Next, they will statistically select the middle 95% of those numbers and designate them as "normal," then they will call the 2.5% that fall above and the 2.5% that fall below that range "abnormal." (In statistics, this is affectionately known as "two standard deviations beyond the mean.") Thus, in the instance of blood glucose, a lab will call anyone who had a value of between 65–100 "normal." Anyone with a value below or above this "normal range" would be called "abnormal." The 65–100 range will represent the values of 95% of the people who had their blood drawn at that lab and is understood to be clustered above and below the "mean" or "average." There is practical validity to this method. For example, most people with a blood glucose less than 100 do not have significant problems. Yet, many people with a glucose above 100 are beginning to have or already have trouble. The higher above 100, the greater the trouble. Experienced physicians and nurse practitioners, however, will start to wonder if a patient who has a blood glucose of 88 for example, isn't giving warnings that they are developing glucose regulating issues. These professionals are aware that healthy young people most often have a blood glucose in the low to mid-70s.

This brings up the issue of "optimal" ranges versus the standard "statistical reference ranges." Exploring this concept further goes beyond the scope of this book. (I do discuss this in depth in our professional training program, www.menopausemethod.com/for-medical-professionals/.)

What is within the scope of this book is that, when treating menopausal women, my best advice is *not* to try to replicate youthful levels of ovarian hormones. Menopausal women can have significant success with lowish dosages of hormones in almost all cases. To the best of my knowledge, considering the potency of hormones and based on the medical, scientific literature, "lowish" is the optimal way to go! Our goal is to alleviate symptoms and optimally support the brain, bones, arteries, muscles, bladder, vagina, etc. Remarkably so, it just doesn't take very much. Certainly not robust or youthful levels.[14.1]

### *Hormonal Dosing Ranges: Individual Variation*

There will be individual variations of dosages from one woman to the next. This individual variability is based upon:

- *Sensitivity.* Women vary as to how sensitive they are to anything they are given. Some women only need a "tiny" amount of hormones because they are so sensitive to medication dosages and many other things.

- *Early life, general hormone levels, and balance.* Some women have robust estrogen levels when they are young and are accustomed to them. Other women have relatively low estrogen levels but have robust amounts of progesterone. Androgen variation plays into this as well. We sometimes gravitate towards treatment levels and balances based on these early-life hormonal patterns. They do not require a special program design: titration of dosages will most often lead to symptom relief.

- *Preference.* Some women prefer less or more of something.

- *Cognitive decline.* There is evidence that in some cases of cognitive decline, higher doses of estrogen than those adequate for bone or vaginal health are required.[14.2]

On rare occasion, a woman will test her hormone levels with the 24-hour urine test when she is in her twenties, healthy and "normal." I do find it interesting to have these youthful values when considering the details of her hormone dosages during menopause. Interesting, yes. Necessary, no... as we aim to fall shy of prescribing youthful hormone levels.

*Hormonal Testing: Thyroid and Adrenals*

It can be difficult to balance the ovarian hormones if there is significant adrenal or thyroid depletion. Thyroid assessment is best accomplished by clinical symptoms, physical examination signs, and blood testing. I find it important to test blood levels of TSH, free T4, free T3, and reverse T3 to have sufficient information. Adrenal hormones are best assessed through the 24-hour urine hormone test and, at times, by additional neurotransmitter testing to assess adrenaline. It can be difficult to achieve menopausal goals with hormones if the thyroid and adrenals are not addressed concurrently.

*Hormonal Testing: Time to Test*

Once again, there are logistics involved in urine testing:

- A full 24-hour collection is required.

- If a woman is regularly menstruating, we will select the day that is three-quarters of the way through her cycle. For example, if she has a 28-day cycle, we would collect on day 19, 20, or 21, counting day one as the first day of menstrual flow. This is the "mid-luteal" phase, halfway between mid-cycle and the end of the cycle. At this time, we can get optimal information about both estrogen and progesterone as they both have simultaneous peaks in levels at this time, as can be seen in Figure 14d.

Figure 14d.

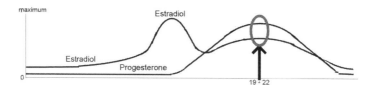

The Time to Test a Regularly Menstruating Woman

- Testing is rarely called for if a woman's periods have become irregular, as the results can be confusing to evaluate.

- If menstruation has ceased for at least several months, it does not matter what day we choose to test. Yet again, as I have mentioned, it is most commonly preferable to test after hormone balance is achieved through treatment.

- Prior to treatment, a menopausal woman's estrogen levels will be too low to assess the quality of the estrogen metabolites.

- The 24-hour urine collection is not an optimal method of testing if there is significant liver or kidney disease.

## *Hormonal Testing: More on Types of Testing*

I would like to elaborate on this subject, which I introduced earlier in this chapter. Testing the blood or saliva for hormones is preferred by many practitioners. Both of these methods definitely have their advocates. There are advantages and disadvantages to all methods, but I prefer not to use blood or saliva testing during perimenopause or menopause for several reasons:

- Precise protocols during saliva collection are crucial for the accuracy and reproducibility of test results; however, they are not uniformly adhered to during collection. Thus, saliva testing is more accurate in a highly controlled research setting.

- Saliva is not a fluid that is part of the normal physiological, hormonal circuitry.

- The amounts of ovarian hormones in the saliva are very small and a fraction of that found in the blood or urine. Therefore, these hormones are technically more difficult to measure.

- During menopause, the ovarian hormones are present in even smaller amounts compared to those of a younger woman. Because of this, the hormones are even more difficult to test in the saliva.

- Only the adrenal hormones, DHEA and cortisol, are present in relatively larger amounts. Consequently, they are easier to test in the saliva.

- I have seen discrepancies in the results of concurrent testing with saliva and urine, with the clinical picture correlating to the urine test only.

- As I mentioned earlier, blood testing is very dependent on the time of collection in evaluating a woman being treated with hormones in menopause, which makes it impractical as an assessment tool.

Saliva testing can be very useful for testing estradiol and progesterone levels in a younger woman where the quantities of these hormones are ample. In questions of fertility, samples can be conveniently collected every three days. This helps us understand hormonal balance throughout the menstrual cycle and reveals if ovulation is taking place, or not.

For thoroughness, I will include four other facts regarding blood testing. This information is important to consider when testing adrenal cortisol levels, selecting a lab, and choosing the proper time for your blood draw:

- First, it is often easier to obtain a sample of blood than urine. On the other hand, a 24-hour urine hormone test sample collection is done entirely at and shipped from home. There is no need to travel to an office to have blood drawn.

- Second, normal fasting morning blood cortisol can be misleading. It is not uncommon for adrenal glands, even when "fatigued," to be able to produce adequate first morning cortisol, yet not have the oomph to produce adequate cortisol for the remainder of the day. A more definitive *blood* test for adrenal cortisol can be done by a provocative challenge which involves the injection of the pituitary hormone ACTH. In this case, an initial reference blood collection is taken, followed by the injection of ACTH, and then followed by a second blood collection. A healthy gland will show an increase of cortisol after the stimulation by the injection of ACTH. A "tired" gland will not demonstrate such a post injection rise in cortisol.

- Third, almost any common lab can provide accurate results for a blood FSH or LH, but it requires a specialty reference lab to provide a trustworthy, accurate analysis of estradiol and progesterone levels. This has to do with the method the lab is using; commonly, older methods are still being used. Also, I have written earlier that the major obstacle for blood estrogen and progesterone assessment comes when trying to assess levels in a menopausal woman who is receiving treatment (see the next bullet point).

• And fourth, when trying to follow hormone levels with blood and saliva testing in women who are taking hormones, we must be very specific about the time of day that we test and consistently retest at the same time. The reason there is time specificity is that hormones, administered by any route, will reach their peak in the blood and then taper off over time, as shown earlier in Figure 14c. The blood or saliva test result is completely influenced by the time you took your hormones in relationship to the time of the blood draw or saliva collection. This is not a problem when assessing a full 24-hour urine and is another reason why I prefer this latter method.

*Sex Hormone Binding Globulin: SHBG*

Once again, a blood test that is recommended in The Menopause Method is the sex hormone binding globulin (SHBG). Every patient gets this test as part of their initial blood profile. It is an interesting one! Ovarian steroid hormones and all adrenal cortical hormones (androgens and corticosteroids) are fat-soluble: they do not dissolve in water. Hmm! Thus, they are not able to travel in the blood stream in a dissolved form, as glucose can. Fat-soluble hormones have to be "bound" and "carried" by "transport" proteins. SHBG is one of these transporters. It is also interesting that a protective mechanism exists if the body senses that steroid hormone levels have gotten too high: the body produces more binding proteins, such as SHBG to bind up the excessive amounts. As an example, let us consider young women who are prescribed birth control pills and are thereby given additional estrogen and an artificial progestin at a time in their lives when they are producing the maximum amount of internal estrogen and progesterone that they will ever make. Their bodies will register the excessive estrogen levels and, often enough, as a means of protection, SHBG will increase to bind the excessive estrogen. This often leads to a simultaneous increased binding of testosterone which is also bound by SHBG. This excessive binding of testosterone in a young woman taking birth control pills often reduces her libido!

Here is yet another quirk in the department of not-common-but-unpleasant occurrences. There is the occasional situation where a woman goes into menopause with the usual very low levels of estrogens and progesterone, yet her SHBG level is elevated! What the heck? Where in the world did this come from? We fully expect to see an elevated SHBG in a woman who has been treated with an excessive amount of ovarian hormones for menopause, but not in a woman who had super-low levels of these hormones prior to any hormone treatment. In a woman who actually has an elevated SHBG prior to treatment, our Menopause Method Questionnaire commonly reveals that she happens to have taken the birth control pill in her youth and often enough, but not always, took it for a number of years. Usually, when a woman stops taking the BCP, the SHBG will gradually return to normal levels. But again, not always! In some cases, the SHBG elevates and remains elevated even though she stopped taking the BCP years or even decades ago.

A significant elevation of SHBG can occur in a menopausal woman treated with excessive estrogens, testosterone, and even excessive thyroid hormones. This can lead to remarkable challenges in dose determination: the more hormones you take (if excessive), the more you bind, and the symptoms of insufficiency persist! I can tell you that technically, this can be a "bear" to rectify. It is achievable, but it sometimes requires medication to accomplish. The moral of the story: avoid an overdose of any of these hormones!

*Hormonal Testing: More About Thyroid Testing*

Traditional thyroid blood tests are valuable for uncovering thyroid disease, yet they are limited using the typical interpreting criteria when it comes to revealing a "tired" thyroid gland producing less than optimal thyroid hormones. All glands can "tire" or "fatigue." If excessive demands are made on them by an overly utilized biological stress response in your classic "fight-or-flight, saber-toothed tiger" situation, the glands can keep up with the excessive demand for a while. At a certain point, however, they can no longer sustain huge production demands and slip into a phase of chronic hormonal underproduction, so-called "glandular fatigue."

If a different interpretation criterion is applied to thyroid test results, more can be learned and utilized from the tests. For example, a common laboratory reference range for thyroid stimulating hormone (TSH)—a hormone that is produced by the pituitary gland, located at the base of the brain, to stimulate the thyroid gland to produce thyroid hormones—is 0.5–4.5. A TSH test result of 3, under traditional interpretation guidelines, would be considered "normal." However, in practical terms, a TSH above 2 could represent a pituitary gland that is efforting more than usual to stimulate a thyroid gland to produce more hormone. This will occur if the brain/pituitary receives information that a less-than-optimal amount of thyroid hormone is circulating about. With a TSH of 3, coupled with symptoms and signs of thyroid function decline, one might have a patient do a "clinical trial" and try a small dose of thyroid hormone treatment to see if greater energy and well-being was achieved. And of course, that dose can be titrated upwards to discover an optimal dose, or, conversely, treatment can be discontinued if symptoms and/or signs of excessive thyroid hormone levels develop. For many reasons, functional thyroid hormone deficiency—thyroid hormone levels that appear within the normal range yet seem insufficient because of symptoms of hypothyroidism, such as tiredness, constipation, and other symptoms—is rampant in the United States. This all makes sense: over time, an excessive, suboptimal response to fight-or-flight stress depletes all relevant glandular hormone production and hormone levels, certainly including the thyroid gland.

The additional blood test results of free T4, free T3, and reverse T3 can help clarify need. For example, a common reference range for free T3 is 2.0–4.4. If a patient's test result is 2.4, it will fall within the reference range. Yet, younger healthy folks have a free T3 level that is commonly 3.0–3.2. A value of 2.4 might correlate with functional hypothyroid hints, such as less energy, slower bowels, and a newfound sense of feeling colder than usual. A trial of thyroid treatment, in my opinion, is called for.

Thyroid, like all hormones, is potent! Too much thyroid dosage often results in experiencing a jittery feeling, the sensation of having drunk too much coffee, as well as having an increased pulse rate, feeling heart palpitations, experiencing tremors, etc. Regardless, if a patient takes thyroid medication and has symptom relief, then six weeks after the dosage levels are clinically determined, the thyroid blood test panel should be repeated to confirm that thyroid levels are optimal.

I always instruct my patients to go into the lab early in the morning and having fasted from the preceding midnight.

If a patient is taking thyroid hormones, they too should be omitted prior to blood draw. As a final note, although thyroid is testable on 24-hour urine hormone test panels, various technical issues in testing thyroid by this method have led me to prefer blood testing for thyroid.

*Hormonal Testing: Adrenal Glands*

Although severe adrenal disease can be revealed by blood tests, non-severe yet significant functional adrenal fatigue may not be detected by simple blood testing. Adrenal hormone secretion can fluctuate over a 24-hour period. Again, one can be misled with a normal morning blood cortisol level: the adrenals may be in good enough shape to produce a normal level overnight (as assessed in a morning blood draw) yet be too "fatigued" to maintain production all day. An afternoon blood sampling for cortisol, which is logistically cumbersome to obtain, could reveal a low cortisol level in this case. The ACTH challenge test can also reveal hypoadrenalcorticism; however, it is costly and logistically cumbersome. Adrenal corticosteroids and androgens are wonderfully assessed in the 24-hour urine hormone test. Adrenal DHEA and cortisol levels can be assessed by salivary testing, for which four samples are obtained at different times of the day.

Adrenal adrenaline production can best be determined by neurotransmitter testing.

I believe at this juncture, although I have not exhausted the topics and details of hormonal testing, I have given you enough information to consider. Once again, there are advantages and disadvantages to all methods. I definitely have my strong preferences. The knowledge, interest, and experience of the individual practitioner is crucial to the choices he or she makes about the methods of testing and the selection of the laboratory.

For the sake of your biochemical entertainment, or if you should ever have the 24-hour urine hormone test performed, I am including (without further explanation) a rather complete biochemical road map of the steroid hormones you may come to know and love (Figure 14e).

## A Final Note About Dosages and Testing

No matter what transdermal hormone preparation you use—organic oils, gels, or creams—and no matter what

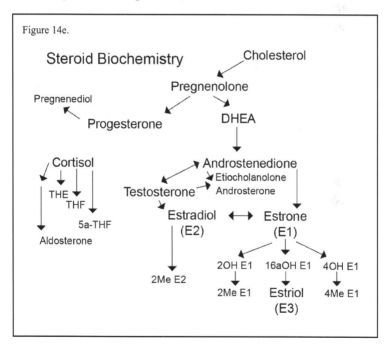

Figure 14e.

**Steroid Biochemistry**

dosage, strength and ratio (for Bi-Est), the most import-ant thing I want you to remember is that when you have stabilized on your regimen, it is *imperative* that you do the

24-hour urine hormone test. Because women vary so much in their ability to absorb any hormone that is applied to the skin, what matters most is what makes it into the body. I find that *only* the 24-hour urine hormone test can accurately detect this. I have treated women with what I was concerned were high dosages of Bi-Est, only to see that their test results were in the optimal range, or even below, of estrogens tested. Vice versa, I have treated women with what I thought were doses too low to help them, only to see test results that showed they were in the optimal range!

Oh my. This has been the third time I have repeated the above paragraph! What the heck! Well, this is because I believe this information is extremely important. Our Menopause Method seeks to reduce risk to as close to zero as possible. None of us are immune from risk, not even from the most challenging of illnesses that exist. As I have discussed, it is my belief that cancer has a multitude of causes, and replenishing with bio-identical hormones is not one of them. (Actually, studies show reduced risk. See Chapter Three: "Risks and Benefits," and the associated articles in Appendix B.) However, a strong case has been made for not treating with supraphysiologic dosages of estrogen.[14.3]

We also know that in the days when conjugated equine estrogens (CEEs) were by far the most prevalent treatment, many women were on excessive dosages, as evidenced by breast tenderness. It was not possible to test for CEEs. Women often enough stayed on excessive dosages for years. And in general, these women did just fine. Yet, there is no reason for excessive dosages, and, in my opinion, the absolute best way to detect them is by 24-hour urine hormone testing.

# Chapter Fifteen

# Patient Assessment: Fundamental Female Evaluations

*Female Exams: The Basics*

There are fundamentals in female medicine for which there are no substitutes. These include:

- Breast self-exams
- Periodic breast and pelvic exams performed by an experienced physician or nurse practitioner
- Mammography
- Thermography
- Transvaginal ultrasound

*Breast Self-Exam*

The information below was copied from the National Breast Cancer Foundation website, Breast Self-Exam: www.nationalbreastcancer.org/breast-self-exam.

Once a month…

1. In the Shower

- Using the pads of your fingers, move around your entire breast in a circular pattern moving from the outside to the center, checking the entire breast and armpit area. Check both breasts each month feeling for any lump, thickening, or hardened knot. Notice any changes and get lumps evaluated by your healthcare provider.

2. In Front of a Mirror

- Visually inspect your breasts with your arms at your sides. Next, raise your arms high overhead.

- Look for any changes in the contour, any swelling, or dimpling of the skin, or changes in the nipples. Next, rest your palms on your hips and press firmly to flex your chest muscles. Left and right breasts will not exactly match—few women's breasts do, so look for any dimpling, puckering, or changes, particularly on one side.

3. Lying Down

- When lying down, the breast tissue spreads out evenly along the chest wall. Place a pillow under your right shoulder and your right arm behind your head. Using your left hand, move the pads of your fingers around your right breast gently in small circular motions covering the entire breast area and armpit.

- Use light, medium, and firm pressure. Squeeze the nipple; check for discharge and lumps. Repeat these steps for your left breast.

And, I would like to include these valuable tips from Eugene Shippen, M.D.: apply oil or soap to your hands (you will feel more) and examine your breasts; take care to feel the depression right behind your nipple.

### Breast Health

I hold prevention as an underlying focus and goal in medicine. Serious illness has an element of mystery to it. I am aware that we are all vulnerable, and there are no guarantees. Yet, at the same time, there is so much that we can do to live healthily without serious illness. In the world of women's health, preventing breast cancer is a wonderful goal.

## Breast Health

*I would like to make three suggestions for your breast health:* [15.1 - 15.4]

- *Diminish bra wearing time. Medical studies have identified reduced risk is correlated with this habit. This allows for freer circulation of blood as well as the lymphatic drainage fluid in the lymph vessels for the natural removal of metabolic, toxic, and other wastes.*

- *Minimize the use of underwire and compression bras. They are the most obstructive to blood flow and lymphatic drainage and should not be used.*

- *Simple, self-administered breast massage. It can be easily performed while showering or bathing and helps lymphatic drainage in the breasts. Stabilize a breast at the nipple with the fingers of one hand. With the fingers of your other hand, press firmly near the nipple and move out peripherally, continuing to press firmly to the edge of the breast. Repeat this "milking-type" process from center to edge until you have covered the entire area of both breasts. The lymphatic channels are low-pressure drainage vessels. Assisting fluid movement within them by external massage is very beneficial from time-to-time or more frequently if you have breast issues. Again, use soap or lotion.*

Although the vast majority of breast and pelvic exams reveal no problems, occasionally something is uncovered. Ideally, detection occurs at as early a stage of anything adverse as possible, when further evaluation, intervention, and treatment can make a beneficial and crucial difference. Assessment and testing of this nature are important and can be critical.

*Breast Imaging and Breast Health*

- *Mammography*

  I am aware that there is controversy about mammography and that many women are concerned about it. I have a strong opinion on this subject. I will never claim that I am always right. However, I promise to give you my "best shot." Caveat emptor. For many years, I had mixed feelings about mammography and was a major proponent of thermography and breast assessment by the patient or a physician or nurse practitioner. I did in no way dissuade my patients from mammography but did not insist upon strict compliance before prescribing hormones. My attitude has changed: I am now a full-fledged proponent of mammography! I had two patients that had negative self-exams and negative thermograms but were later diagnosed with breast cancer on routine mammograms. These two cancers were caught and treated very early on, which is so beneficial with this disease. For each woman, the art and science of mammography calls for individualizing both her imaging prescriptions and their timing.

  For perimenopausal or menopausal women with no breast issues (e.g., no issues on self-exam, medical exam, mammography, no lumps, no breast tenderness, no increased breast density, no previous fibrocystic issues, no familial risk, etc.), I recommend annual mammograms. If a few negative mammograms are completed, I readily shift to every one and a half years, two years, or even three years.

For women with breast issues, the rate of repeat mammography is most commonly every year yet can be as often as every six months and is rarely more than every year. It is often coupled with breast ultrasound and breast thermography. These women can often be assisted by adjusting hormone dosages and ratios as well as with supplemental iodine and DIM, as per discussions with their medical professional. Other diagnostic procedures such as special genetic testing (e.g., BRCA gene, HER2/neu) are often indicated. The general knowledge regarding mammography and breast health is to individualize diagnostic and treatment protocols, one woman to the next.

- *Breast Ultrasound*
  This is another testing method of merit. Information gained from this non-invasive technique that utilizes a low intensity of energy can reveal a breast abnormality. However, it is not held to be a primary breast imaging screening technique, and it is most commonly used to obtain additional information when a screening mammogram raises a question about a possible breast issue. A radiologist will often suggest or implement this additional test when the mammogram is insufficiently conclusive.

For more information, the American Cancer Society has a good description of breast imaging techniques: visit www.cancer.org/cancer/breast-cancer/screening

- *Breast Thermography*

  This is yet another breast imaging assessment method that can have value. However, I recommend that you proceed with caution. For this screening, a woman stands in front of a heat-sensitive "camera" and a recording of heat patterns is made. Increased heat in a breast can occur when there is decreased lymph and blood flow within and outgoing from the breast tissue. This restricts the outflow of biochemicals produced by breast cell metabolism. It is important that these biochemicals leave the breast and are processed by the liver and kidneys. One example of a biochemical byproduct of metabolism is lactic acid, a buildup of this in the tissues can be irritating and, thus, unhealthy. There are other possibilities as well.

  The main cause of breast lymphatic flow restriction is the use of underwire and compression bras as well as excessive bra use (Figure 15a). Breast health is dependent upon the moment-to-moment movement of unconstrained breasts, the bounce. This action stimulates the passive

Figure 15a.

Effect of Compression and Underwire Bras

with compression & underwire bra

after discontinuing this bra

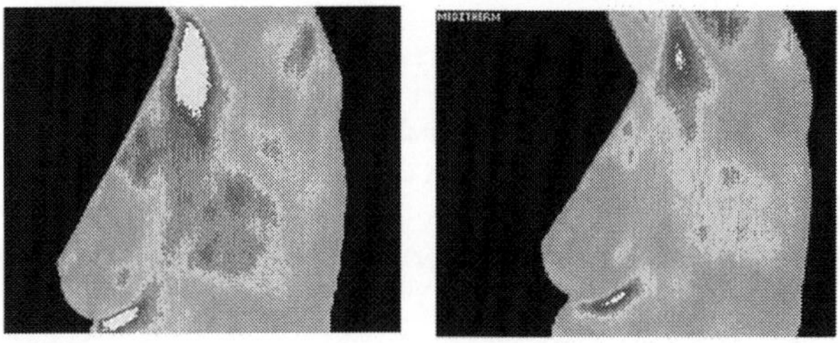

nature of the lymphatic flow, similar to how walking supports lower extremity blood and lymphatic flow.

Increased heat can also result from increased blood circulation to the breast, as in the overstimulation of breast glandular tissue caused by excessive or imbalanced hormones. Likewise, this can be caused by administered hormones. The birth control pills taken by young women are a classic example as they contain estradiol and a progestin: they add hormones to a woman's body when she is producing them at the highest levels of her entire life. In Figure 15b, you can see the thermogram images of a young woman before and after birth control pill usage.

Figure 15b.

Effect of Birth Control Pills on Breast Tissue

before birth control use          6 months after birth control use

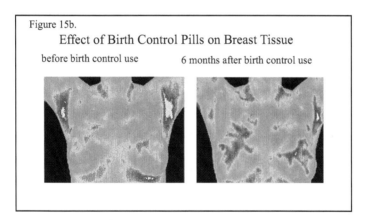

In menopausal women, overtreatment with estrogens or undertreatment with progesterone can be a cause as well. At times, excessive estrogen from other causes can result in the overstimulation of breast glandular tissue.

Excessive estrogen and increased heat can also be caused by:

- Again, the overtreatment of women in menopause with excessive dosages of estrogens is problematic. One of the fundamental objectives of The Menopause Method is to achieve optimal estrogen levels... not too little and not too much. As I mentioned earlier, it doesn't take much! Certainly, it takes less than in young women. In our professional training program, we specifically define the dosages and testing parameters that we consider to be optimal: www.menopausemethod.com.

- Excessive stress. Estrogen will function as an additional stress hormone if need be and will be produced in higher amounts during stressful situations! Wow! Think about that!

- Insufficient progesterone will lead to "estrogen dominance" effects as there will not be adequate progesterone to balance the estrogens.

- Lastly, inflammatory conditions of the breast tissue, such as fibrocystic breast disease as well as types of cancer, are yet another cause of increased heat. Certain types of breast cancer are rapid growing and generate their own increased blood circulation to support that rapid growth. This increased blood flow brings the increased heat. Some of these breast cancers can, therefore, be detected by thermography.

One moral of this story is to reduce the amount of bra wearing in general and eliminate the use of compression and underwire bras. Medical studies have shown reduced incidence of breast cancer in cultures where bra use is minimal to none. Refer to the references cited in Appendix B for information on this important topic.[15.1 - 15.4]

Bra use, meant to address breast "sagging," can diminish the natural uplift of the breasts by the chest muscles. Breasts have no internal musculature support to lift them. Chest pectoral muscles aid in this support. Normal breast bounce helps exercise those pectoral muscles. Bras can be antagonistic to the bounce of the breasts which benefits those muscles. Googling "prevention of sagging breasts" will lead you to many resources on this topic. You can also google "healthy bra" and find even more information and resources.

## *Eliminate compression and underwire bras, reduce bra wear, and you can do great good!*

To see an example of how thermography was a useful tool in our practice, see illustration 15c on page 195. I also discuss this subject in more detail in our training program for professionals, The Menopause Method (www.menopausemethod.com).

I'd like to share a story about one of my patients, B.D. She was in her mid-forties when I first saw her for perimenopausal issues. She had never been pregnant and had longstanding breast issues, which is sometimes the case in women who have never been pregnant. She had chronic breast tenderness and had been diagnosed with fibrocystic breast disease. Mammograms over the years repeatedly demonstrated increased breast density, which is a risk factor for breast cancer. To me, chronic breast tenderness is unacceptable. It speaks to either or both:

- Overstimulation of the breast glandular tissue by hormonal excess or imbalance.
- The possibility of underlying lymphatic drainage issues, inflammation, fibrocystic changes, etc.

  *We are a "no breast tenderness" practice. I will continue to work with the women who have breast tenderness until it is alleviated! It can be alleviated!*

In the case of my patient, B.D., I suggested the following:

- Reducing hormone treatment dosages. Her body had been used to robust estrogen levels, and she had titrated up to higher treatment dosages. These robust, and to me excessive, hormone levels were detected by 24-hour urine hormone testing. B.D. is a woman who is highly committed to her health and went through the gradual process of dose reduction, tolerating the symptoms that eventually alleviated over time and with her diligence.

- Adding iodine to her supplement program. The initial doses were up to 50 mg per day which we intentionally reduced over time to 12.5 mg per day. Iodine can be "magic" in its benefit for women who have breast issues. I so highly recommend it. However, caution must be exercised as excessive iodine can be toxic to the thyroid, for one.[15.5] Periodic monitoring of thyroid function by blood testing of TSH, free T4, free T3, and reverse T3 is crucial.

- Eliminating compression, underwire, and excessive bra use.[15.1 - 15.4]

- Assuring that menopausal progesterone treatment levels were adequate. Annual 24-hour urine hormone tests support this assessment. At one point, we discovered the progesterone dosages and carriers that had served her well in the past no longer produced adequate progesterone levels; undoubtedly, she had developed absorption issues. Monitoring and adjusting dosages and routes of administration have worked quite well in her case.

- Changing her therapy from estradiol to Bi-Est.

We followed her progress by thermography. We also had a major clinical indicator: we did not stop focusing on her situation until all of her breast tenderness, which she'd had for years, had disappeared! See the progression of thermograms over three years in Figure 15c.

Figure 15c.

Resolution of Breast Tenderness Over Years

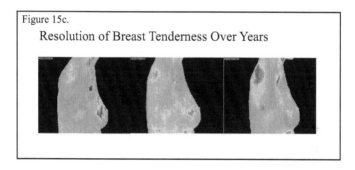

*We are a "no breast tenderness" practice.*
*I will continue to work with the women who*
*have breast tenderness until it is alleviated!*
*It can be alleviated!*

*A Final Word and Caution About*
*Breast Imaging and*
*Thermography in Particular*

*No breast assessment technique is perfect: false negatives (an illness in the breast exists and the imaging technique misses it) and false positives (the image suggests breast pathology and it is not so, as revealed by biopsy or surgery) occur. A disclaimer exists on mammogram reports that states "four to eight percent of breast cancers are missed by X-ray techniques." Thermography, no matter how much one would like to believe that it is the alternative to mammography, has false negatives as well. A reputable thermographer, as I have had the privilege to know, will disclose that to their patients. However, in my opinion, you can encounter enthusiasm for this method that outstrips the method's capability. I have had three cases in my practice that were thermogram false negatives. The first was a mother of two in her thirties that felt a breast lump and chose thermography to evaluate it. She was told it was negative for cancer. She first came to see me after it had progressed and then was diagnosed on a mammogram as a large breast cancer. Surgical and other treatment followed, yet she died within a year of discovery. The second case involved a patient of mine who postponed her mammogram (which I did not know about) because she took false assurance in a negative thermogram. Fortunately, when the small lump persisted, and she decided to go ahead with the mammogram, the cancer was detected and removed at an early stage. The third case involved*

> *a patient who had a thermogram and mammogram at nearly the same time. The thermogram was negative, the mammogram positive, and the cancer was confirmed on surgical removal.*
>
> *Please do not get inappropriately enthusiastic about thermography. I still utilize thermography and appreciate it for its revealing of health compromise in the breasts. I do not recommend it as a cancer screening tool... certainly not the only tool chosen!*

I assert with careful focus on each individual woman's particular issues as they relate to breast health and risk, properly designed screening techniques, which definitely include mammograms, can be implemented for the ultimate benefit of every woman. With that said, mammograms do not necessarily have to be performed annually, in my opinion. Each woman's individual situation will suggest an optimal timing between studies.

### Annual Exam: Breasts, Pelvic, Pap, and Transvaginal Ultrasound (TVUS)

Gynecologists have many other examinations, tests, and treatments that can be very important to your well-being.

For menopausal women taking estrogens, our Menopause Method protocol calls for the following health screenings:

- A complete annual female in-office exam performed by a woman's physician, gynecologist, or nurse practitioner.

- A routine pap smear.

- An assessment of vaginal health during a woman's annual exam. This is crucial for proper menopausal hormone treatment. Why "crucial?" As I have mentioned, a hallmark sign of the many changes that occur in menopause is the atrophying of the vagina. A young vagina is relatively thick, has a multitude of tiny "folds," and it has healthy surface cells that keep the vagina moist and lubricated during sexual intercourse. The vagina of an untreated menopausal woman invariably is thin and dry. Because of this, questioning a patient if she has pain with intercourse or if she must utilize a lubricant product is important and very revealing; women who have pain or who need lubrication have significant vaginal atrophic changes. Treatment will reverse vaginal atrophy and restore a reasonable level of vaginal health with adequate restoration of estrogen levels.

Additionally once again, this is very important for bladder reasons. The tube that empties the urinary bladder opens up into the vagina near its end. That "urethral meatus," as it is known, is part of the vagina and is vulnerable to the atrophic changes of the vagina mucosa. The meatus can be easily irritated and become inflamed, and lead to urinary frequency, urgency, nighttime urination, infections, and, ultimately to the need for padded disposable underwear. This is the result of vaginal atrophy, coupled with the weakening of the muscle, the levator ani, which supports the bladder and often weakens as women lose their androgens.

- Our medical literature is very clear: it takes a minimal amount of treatment with estrogen to restore reasonable vaginal health.[15.6] Also, if the vagina is relatively healthy, there is evidence that dosage levels of estrogen are also sufficient to protect the bones![15.6]

- A yearly uterine transvaginal ultrasound for all women who have not had a hysterectomy. This is to assess the health of the uterine lining in women utilizing hormones. We are looking for a uterine "stripe" that is less than 5 mm in thickness or less than 4 or 3 mm and is "uniform" in thickness without any unusual deformities. Although relatively rare, I have seen cases of uterine cancer. The miracle was that they were detected at a very early stage by transvaginal ultrasound and then treated successfully.

- Because the majority of my menopausal patients have a personal gynecologist, general physician, or nurse practitioner who they see for annual female exams, I instruct them to ask specific questions at the time of that visit. I would like to know, on a scale of one to five (with five being the "highest"), the quality of vaginal health and vaginal atrophy compared to that of a 28-year-old woman. At times, a woman must ask these questions with a certain amount of diplomacy, as physicians and nurse practitioners routinely observe vaginal atrophy in menopausal women. Consequently, they may be reluctant to show concern if a patient is not experiencing vaginal or bladder problems. When asked about vaginal health, they may reply that it is "normal for your age." We ask our patients to respectively probe for clarity regarding vaginal health.

*Bone Density and Bone Health*

Bone health can be assessed by an X-ray procedure known as "bone mineral density." This certainly remains a "gold standard" for evaluation. Bone loss can also be assessed by measuring biochemical breakdown products of the bone that appear in the urine: "pyridinium" and "deoxy-pyridinoline." Also, measuring urine acidity at home can give you clues to excessive body acidity which is relevant to bone loss. I will discuss this subject in further detail in the next chapter.

Chapter Sixteen

# Osteoporosis and Restoration of Bone Health

No discussion about menopause would be complete without addressing the subject of bones. Osteoporosis is bone loss, sometimes mild (osteopenia), sometimes moderate or even severe (osteoporosis). This loss is caused by a gradual leaching out over time of the molecular structure of bone, its minerals, and protein. These minerals and protein are what bones are made of! From that microscopic thinning out, the bones become fragile and are more likely to break. This fragility, coupled with a fall, is often just enough to cause a hip or other bone to fracture all too easily. Osteoporosis has many factors associated with its development, and the loss of ovarian hormones during menopause is surely one of them.

I so clearly remember a lecture in medical school by a gerontologist, a specialist in treating the elderly. He said,

> "You have learned about many diagnoses in your training, all of which can occur in the elderly. But let me tell you what is all too commonly happening with older folks. They have sarcopenia, which is muscle loss so significant that they have trouble rising from a chair as well as standing or walking with stability. Because of this, they can easily fall, and when they do, so often, it is onto osteoporotic bones. From that point on, it is fractures, hospitalization, operations, and if they can make it through this process, rehabilitation and often wheelchairs."

As we examine the causes of and treatments for osteoporosis, we will consider hormones, nutrition, digestion, nutritional supplements, the buffering of excessive body acid, and exercise.

*Hormones and Bone Health*

Bone, at first thought, could seem to be a static tissue. It is not. It is constantly being broken down and rebuilt. The hormones—progesterone, estrogens, testosterone, DHEA, cortisol, and thyroid—play a significant role in bone health. Many women have osteoporosis because of hormone deficiency. Hormones are powerful, and when inadequate, their absence is felt. For example, women who undergo total hysterectomies (surgical removal of the uterus plus both ovaries) have an increased incidence of osteoporosis if they are not treated with ovarian hormones.[16.1] This makes sense as estrogens slow down the activity of cells called osteoclasts, the cells that break down bone![16.2] Progesterone directly and beneficially affects cells called osteoblasts, which lay down new bone.[16.3]

*Nutrition and Bone Health: You Are What You Eat—And What You Digest*

Bone is constructed out of protein and minerals. Because of this, bone renewal is subject to:

- the content and quality of the nutrients in the food that you purchase and eat, as well as;
- your ability to digest this food and assimilate its nutrients.

For example, human height has increased over time and has always had a significant relationship to the quality and quantity of food available. In times and places of low food availability, average height declines, and, it increases when access to food increases.

In the past, soils were richer, and the food was more nutrient dense. Rather affluent people often had the luxury of nutritious diets. Also, people were more physically active and were exposed to fewer toxins. A healthier diet, exercise, and lifestyle, greatly diminishes the risk for osteoporosis and other health problems.

Nowadays, most conventionally produced food in America is grossly low in nutrient content. As early as the 1930s, the United States Senate reported that American soils have mineral deficiencies.[16.4] Agribusiness has aggravated this situation through unhealthy farming methods.

This nutrient content deficiency is the principle reason for the flatter taste of conventional food. I used to wonder why grocery market food did not taste like food! When I was young, my grandparents would take me with them when they would go to pick fresh corn, tomatoes, and other produce from a local farm. The taste of this produce was amazing, as was that of chicken and most everything else! What has happened? Today, food can be as bland as the plastic container in which it is packaged! So, the initial problem concerning bone health can be the poor nutrient content of the food.

There has been "much ado" about "organic" food. Just to set the record straight, all food on the planet Earth was organic from the time humans appeared 200,000 years ago until the 1950s. "Organic" means the food was grown by natural methods on natural soil, free of added chemicals such as herbicides, pesticides, and chemical fertilizers. The farmers who care about these issues continue to grow organic food, as they always have, and a whole new generation of farmers have turned to restoring soils and growing foods organically.

Again, I want to give you my "best shot" about nutrition, much in the way I like to follow the automobile care guidelines that my auto mechanic does for his car. Likewise, to give you an idea of the nutritional guidelines that I have followed in my personal life for decades, I'll summarize them for you. These guidelines are not only based on my taste preference — I, like so many, love food — but from decades of research into nutrition:

- Organic, organic, organic. For home use, we only purchase organic. The organic world is not perfect as there is variation in quality and freshness to be sure, but it is usually as good as it gets.

- When purchasing eggs, dairy, poultry, and meat, pay careful attention to how the animals are raised and fed (many markets today specify these details).

  o Meats are ideally "free range"... animals are raised roaming green pastures. They are not living in cattle concentration camps, known as "feedlots," penned in all their lives.

  o They are grass-fed and "finished." They are not primarily fed grain and soy products, which increase their fat content, and in a way, that is not healthy for us.

- In restaurants, and when I travel, I do the best I can and don't upset myself if the food choices are not optimal.

- Consume whole and fresh foods.

- Minimize boxes, bottles, and cans — processed foods.

I'd like to put in a special "plug" for farmers' markets. This is as close to "farm-to-table" as we can get. They often have a significant number of organic growers. The farmers and their helpers can be quite fun to deal with. *The prices cannot be beat!* And, here you are, out walking in the fresh air amongst the people of your community... my goodness, it can be people watching at its best! I confess that our farmer's market is one of the highlights of my week.

Bone health is also subject to your ability to digest, absorb, and assimilate nutrients that are present in food. Digestion is paramount. What you eat is one thing. What you digest is another! Protein and minerals require significant and sophisticated digestive power.

Digestion begins with chewing; many people rush through their meals without adequately chewing their food. Chewing breaks down the food into tiny particles which is so essential for the subsequent enzyme and acid stages of digestion. It's a physics principle, "surface area to solvent," that scientifically describes what is common sense: the smaller the particle, the easier it is to dissolve. Picture two glasses of acid standing side by side. Picture two marbles, one of them whole and the other crushed to a fine powder. Picture dropping the whole marble into one of the glasses and all of the powdered marble into the second glass. Which will dissolve first: the whole marble or the powdered marble?

The kind of tininess we are medically looking for begins with thorough chewing. Once again, your mother or your grandmother were right when they told you to "chew your food!" You can learn more on this topic from our medical educational project: www.iwonderdoctor.com/pages/digestion.

Not so commonly known is that natural and fresh foods contain digestive enzymes to assist with their own digestive process. Most modern, non-organic foods, and especially those that are not fresh, are grossly deficient in these enzymes. When an apple falls to the ground, we say it "rots." Not true: the impact of the fall breaks open some of the apple's surface cells that then let loose with their digestive enzymes. Enzymatic digestion then begins and ends with the apple turning to mush... through digestion!

Additionally, if a person has experienced long-term stress, it becomes less and less likely that sufficient hydrochloric acid will be available for digestion. This powerful stomach acid is necessary for the digestion of protein and minerals in food. It is easy to understand that in the biology of the stress response, powerful mobilizing hormones such as adrenaline and cortisol are produced in abundance. It is not so easy to understand why hydrochloric acid is produced and excreted during the stress response, whether needed for digestion or not. For whatever reason, the repeated excessive production of hydrochloric acid ultimately, in the long run, leads to reduced amounts of it being produced. Thus, less is available for digestion as we age. Additionally, as we grow older, we have fewer and fewer digestive enzymes (again, probably due to previous stress), which are necessary to further digest the elements of food. Hence, our ability to digest minerals and protein is diminished and, as a result, our bones can be compromised.

Absorption is yet another facet of digestion that affects the bones. For a variety of reasons, intestinal issues are common.

Many problems result from hidden infections, often not readily apparent, of the intestinal tract that are caused by unbeneficial bacteria and yeast, etc. These critters are unacceptable to our immune system. The interaction between our immune system and the infection can lead to low-grade inflammation of our intestinal lining. This can lead to gut surface absorption problems, increased intestinal permeability ("leaky gut"), "food allergy" and, ultimately, to compromised absorption and reduced assimilation of nutrients. Once again, this will result in a reduction of proteins and minerals that are available for the bone rebuilding process, among other things.

### *Excessive Cellular Acidity*

Overall, excessive acid in our cells is another important factor to consider in osteoporosis. Here, I am referring to the acid that can be produced in our cells and may become excessive from a variety of causes. This acidity is quite different from the stomach acid related to digestion.

All food is eventually broken down into tiny molecules and ends up in the cells of our body to be biochemically transformed in a process called "metabolism." One result of metabolic biochemistry is the internal cellular production of acid or alkaline biochemicals. All foods are known to ultimately have either an acid outcome or an alkaline outcome. Proteins such as meat primarily have an acidic effect. On the other hand, vegetable metabolism mainly has an alkaline effect.

Our bodies are very careful and precise in the regulation of acidity: we do not function well if our cells become too acidic. When people with diabetes end up in emergency rooms, it is usually because of excessive acidity. In their case, however, it developed from problems related to diabetes and not from regular food metabolic processing. The common and widespread excess acidity that we find in many people is no way as severe or of such immediate threat as it is in diabetic acidosis. However, the bottom line with too much cellular acidity is that it needs to be neutralized or "buffered" — a process that reduces the acidity overall. In the long run, problems resulting from excessive acidity can be significant.

The demand to buffer acid is high because excessive acidity can injure many of our essential internal biochemicals. Our most immediate buffering mechanism combines the excess acid with bicarbonate present in our blood and produces carbon dioxide, which we then exhale from our lungs. When this primary mechanism is overloaded from excessive acidity, we utilize a backup buffering system. In this case, our body buffers the excessive acid by combining the acid with minerals and other bicarbonates.

Where does our body acquire the necessary minerals and bicarbonates to do this type of buffering? The minerals and bicarbonates come from where they are present in greatest abundance: our bones! Our precious bone calcium, magnesium, trace minerals, and bicarbonates will be extracted from the bone if need be to address the biological priority of buffering excessive acid.

How do we get too much cellular acid? Food and stress are the two major sources. Once again, during the biochemical processing of

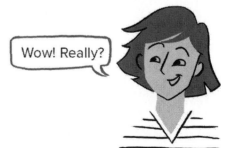

Wow! Really?

all foods, on a cellular level, there is the possibility that acid can be produced. Recall, this is more probable with some foods than others. Acid formation results from the cellular "burning" of protein derived from animal food sources and, especially, excessive dietary intake of animal protein. The other, and often more significant, producer of excessive cellular acidity is the biochemistry that results from stress!

Not only does stress result in an excessively acidic metabolism, a robust secretion of cortisol (a premier stress hormone) has the "side effect" of causing the excessive dissolution of bones! Once again, we encounter a consequence of stress. Stress negatively affects bone health just as it affects hormonal health.

In our office, we ask anyone with diminished bone density to test* their urine for three days with acid-testing strips. We ask that they record the time and the acidity of *every* urination. Testing all urine is necessary to truly understand the pattern of acidity. If their urine results are too acidic (<7), we make dietary and other adjustments to buffer this excessive acid and, therefore, conserve bone minerals!

***Address the biological priority of buffering excessive acid so that our precious calcium, magnesium, trace minerals, and bicarbonates are not extracted from the bone***

* Urine pH (acid testing) paper in the correct pH range can be purchased from online vendors. The range needs to be at least 5.5 to 8.0. Search for "pH test tape."

*Assessing Bone Health*

The "gold standard" for accessing bone health is the bone mineral density X-ray test. Dense bones show up well on X-ray, and bone density can be measured. Bones that have lost a significant amount of minerals and protein appear much lighter.

A common bone mineral density report is seen in Figure 16a. This illustration shows an image of the hip. Also, rou-

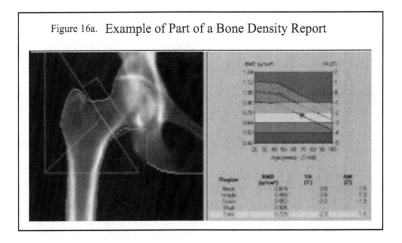

Figure 16a. Example of Part of a Bone Density Report

tinely included in this test is an image of the lumbar spine. These represent two important regions to assess. Hip fracture is all too common, a consequence of significant osteoporosis.

Whenever I see a bone density report that reveals osteoporosis or osteopenia, one of the questions I have is whether or not the bones are *continuing* to lose minerals and proteins. It is common that the significant bone loss took place in the past and is not vigorously or actively occurring presently. An example of that would be a woman who went into menopause at the age of 45 and did not receive treatment with ovarian hormones. By the time she is 55, the likelihood of her developing significant osteopenia or even osteoporosis is quite high. However, the majority of that bone loss could have taken place in the first five years of her having dramatically reduced estrogen levels. I want to know if there is still an active bone loss. If there is, it calls for additional treatment measures.

Bone metabolism has biochemical byproducts. When the bone breaks down, these byproducts end up in the blood stream and are eventually excreted in the urine. During active bone turnover, we see increased levels of these byproducts in the urine. An easy-to-perform test will check for these metabolites. Two common tests we request are deoxypyridinoline crosslinks (DPD) (it took me years to pronounce this correctly!) and N-telopeptides (NTx). In Figure 16b, we show an example of a test result. In this case, the patient is registering excessive amounts of metabolites in her urine, indicating that bone loss is actively occurring and not just a thing of the past.

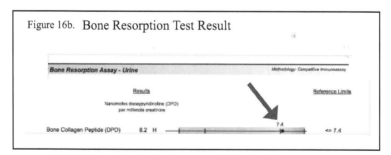

Figure 16b. Bone Resorption Test Result

## Assessing Bone Health: Additional Testing

As you are probably aware, vitamin D plays a significant role in bone health. Vitamin D levels are readily determined by a blood test from a medical laboratory. The test that should be ordered is "25-hydroxy vitamin D."

The reference ranges tend to be wide. In women with bone loss, I like to see levels brought up to at least 60 ng/ml. These levels are invariably achieved through supplementation with a high-quality vitamin D3 supplement. Common dosages are 1,000 IU, 2,000 IU, and 5,000 IU.

Caution with vitamin D dosage is required because, like all fat-soluble vitamins, if taken in excess, it can accumulate in the body and have adverse consequences. I highly recommend:

- All women with bone loss should have their vitamin D level tested.

- Vitamin D should be prescribed in recommended dosages by a knowledgeable health professional.

- After one month of treatment, retest to assess if serum vitamin D levels are in the range of 60–80 ng/ml (not higher or lower).

There are further tests and replenishing that are possible and important, including these:

- Mineral levels such as magnesium and trace minerals can be tested. This is done in traditional and specialty labs that assess red blood cell, plasma, and whole blood levels. This is necessary to get accurate results.

- Amino acid levels can also be tested by specialty laboratories. These levels and balance are important and are basic indicators of how well proteins are being digested.

- Of course, you have heard of supplementing with adequate calcium in the form of nutritional supplements. It is important to know the type of calcium as it can come in forms that are challenging to digest and assimilate.

One such form is calcium carbonate, which could be derived from limestone or oyster shell. This was the most common calcium in the past and is very inexpensive.

The challenging information that you need 1400 mg of calcium per day is derived from the old-fashioned way of reporting the weight of the whole molecule of calcium carbonate in milligrams. Up-to-date calcium recommendations speak to the more digestible and assimilatable calciums, for example, calcium hydroxyapatite, citrate, or malate. The recommendation is for 400 mg per day of the elemental calcium derived from calcium hydroxyapatite. Nowadays, manufacturers of quality supplements report the amount of elemental calcium available from their calcium combination supplements. It has been stated that we are not capable of assimilating more than 400 mg of elemental calcium per day.

- A similar situation exists for magnesium. It is available in many forms, from the very difficult to absorb and assimilate, magnesium hydroxide (and cheap), to the high-quality magnesium glycinate (and more expensive).

- Also to be considered in a supplement program for bone health are vitamin K2, silicon, and trace minerals.

Testing is also available to assess digestion and intestinal health. Many health professionals who are knowledgeable in functional medicine are familiar with the excellent stool labs and tests. Shy of esoteric testing, digestion can be evaluated by the following symptoms that may appear when digestion is compromised:

- Diminishing quality of hair and nails.

- Excessive burping when eating.

- Excessive gas from the other end.

- A feeling of being "full" or bloated long after a meal.

- Stools that float on the surface are an indicator that fats are not being digested properly.

- Stools that sink to the bottom are an indicator that minerals are not being digested adequately.

- Stools that are too soft are an indicator of several possibilities, including poor digestion, too rapid a "transit time," or from an infection or inflammation.

- Stools that are too hard (and normally were not) are an indicator that you may not be drinking sufficient water or digesting protein adequately. Undigested protein is sticky, like glue, causing stools to be hard.

- "GERD" or "acid stomach burn." What appears to be excessive stomach acidity can be quite deceiving and actually represent insufficient stomach acid! Robust stomach acid is necessary for the maintenance of a germ-free stomach. When stomach acid levels decline, infections and thus inflammation can occur in the stomach, which leads to hypersensitivity of the stomach lining to its own stomach acid. Consequently, discomfort or pain results… even if that acid production is reduced below adequate levels. Some (not all) people with "acid indigestion" actually need supplemental acid to heal the stomach! This may be the reason that some people with stomach problems benefit greatly from apple cider vinegar, as vinegar is a weak acid. This topic is really the province of a skilled health professional who is knowledgeable in the complexity of these issues. There certainly are incidents where "acid blocking" medications are needed. To learn more, visit www.iwonderdoctor.com/pages/digestion.

*Exercise and Bone Strength*

Exercise is vital for building strong bones. Surgeons, for several reasons, encourage patients to get up out of bed sometimes long before they may feel like doing so. Likewise, all physicians are especially concerned about patients who are bedridden for extended lengths of time. One of the main reasons is that being inactive can absolutely lead to bone loss, sometimes severe. This excessive calcium leaching from the bones can lead to excessive calcium in the urine and even to kidney stones. At times, it can also lead to the development of very large urinary tract calcifications.

The good news is that substantial physical movement throughout the day can assist in maintaining and healing the bones. Walking, for example, is terrific. It turns out that exercises such as walking that involve impact are crucial. Every time your foot "hits" the ground, a mini-impact that is felt all the way up your legs, thighs, hips, and spine occurs. That impact is crucial. Riding a bike, exercising on an elliptical machine, and swimming are certainly great for the muscles and heart—but are not that beneficial for the bones. Walking on a treadmill does have that step-by-step impact. Would you like to help your bones heal? Walk, walk, walk.

*Summary of an Osteoporosis Treatment Program*

Below are some helpful guidelines for maintaining and building strong bones:

- Hormone replenishing is at the core of addressing bone loss, that is for sure.
- The foundation of nutrition is based upon food that is organic, organic, organic!
  - Protein intake needs to be generous but not excessive. The amount required can vary according to metabolic individuality: some of us do better on a plant-based diet, others do better on a diet that is more robust in protein (including animal protein), and others "fall" somewhere in between. Nutritionists knowledgeable in this field can assist you.
  - Body acidity issues can call for modifications in protein intake.
- Digestion needs to be augmented with proper chewing. This one act of slowing down and thoroughly chewing your food will assist digestion as much as anything.
  - Also, at times, digestive enzyme supplements can be added. Taking one to four capsules per meal can be beneficial and usually should be taken at the end of a meal.
  - When tolerated, we also add hydrochloric acid in the form of a dietary supplement called "betaine hydrochloride." A few minutes into the meal (to mimic stomach acid production), take one to four capsules. For more information on supplements and digestion, please visit www.iwonderdoctor.com/pages/digestion.
- Intestinal absorption and infection issues may need to be addressed.
- Supplement with vitamins and minerals.

- ○ This begins with a high-quality multiple vitamin/mineral formulation.

- ○ Additional mineral supplements can be added, emphasizing quality supplements in an assimilable form, such as calcium hydroxyapatite or calcium citrate (e.g., 400 mg elemental calcium) and magnesium glycinate (e.g., 300–600 mg elemental magnesium).

- ○ Additional trace minerals such as boron and others can be helpful.

- ○ Vitamins D and K relate strongly to bone health. (See the previous details regarding vitamin D supplementation.)

- Monitor urine acidity. If excessive (frequently below seven and even less beneficial, below six), pH levels can be adjusted if need be with diet modifications. If that is not sufficient, supplements designed to buffer excessive acid are available.

- Weight bearing and "impact" exercises such as walking are essential.

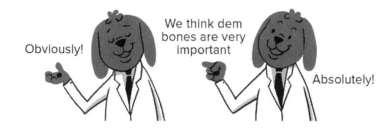

217

Chapter Seventeen

# Weight Issues in Menopause

Weight gain can be a common issue for women during menopause. It is a complex subject* that is influenced by many variables. More is understood about weight gain and loss than ever before. Gone are the days of singular reliance upon calories in/calories out, calorie counting, and low-fat diets. Many factors can intersect during a woman's forties and fifties. These include the following:

- Excessive intake of carbohydrates, especially simple carbohydrates (the worst case: almost anything sweet).

- Diminished ability to physiologically manage carbohydrates (glucose/insulin regulating issues).

- Increased insulin resistance caused by excessive carbohydrates, adrenaline, cortisol, glucagon, and by diminished estrogens.

- Diminished hormones: of course, estrogen, progesterone, and soon, if not already, testosterone and DHEA, as well as the possibility of lowish thyroid levels.

- Decreasing metabolic rate of caloric "burn" caused by a variety of reasons, including excessive calorie restriction and hormonal decline.

- An exaggerated response to stress that triggers excessive stress hormones, thus blood glucose elevations and insulin resistance.

* Author's note: hold onto your seatbelts. This chapter may only be for the physiologically enchanted amongst you. You could jump to the end of the chapter for a summary.

- Insufficient physical activity.

- Reduced neurotransmitter levels, especially serotonin and the catecholamines (e.g., adrenaline and noradrenaline), leading to an excessive appetite.

- Nutrient depletion in non-organic foods, resulting in additional hunger for missing nutrients. Consequently, we graze through and consume additional food, thus calories, in a quest to meet minimum nutritional needs—especially those of depleted minerals and vitamins.

- Eating to "quiet" your uncomfortable emotions or to fill any void you have for what you feel is missing.

- Other causes, such as an intestinal yeast infection.

### *Carbohydrates, Glucose, Insulin, Adrenaline, and Cortisol*

One of the more common causes of unwanted weight gain is the excessive intake of carbohydrates. Because fat deposition is so obvious when someone gains extra weight, there is a generalized "fear of fat." Surprise: more often, at the root of unwanted weight gain, of body fat accumulation, is the *excessive intake of carbohydrates.* Carbohydrates can be converted into fat in the body, and if more carbohydrates are eaten than are needed, any leftovers *will* be converted into fat. This fat is "stored away for a rainy day" when food may not be available.

As you may know, pure food consists of carbohydrates, proteins, fats, vitamins, minerals, and water. Carbohydrates are comprised, in essence, of long "chains" of a type of sugar molecule known as "glucose." These chains easily break down to glucose by a simple digestive process.

Digested foods are assimilated into our bodies and then "metabolized." Metabolism is an exquisitely orchestrated and complex biochemical process that:

- produces energy, whereby food is chemically transformed ("burned"), and energy and heat are released;

- produces essential biochemicals, substances, and structures such as enzymes, hormones, cell nuclei, bones, muscles, and so much more;

- eliminates waste, for instance, the "waste" byproducts of a myriad of chemical reactions are eliminated.

The ultimate digestive breakdown products of carbohydrates, proteins, and fats (i.e., glucose, amino acids, and fatty acids) are the fuels for all metabolic energy production. Vitamins and minerals also play an assisting role to all of the biochemical reactions. All of these basic derivatives of food are the biochemical building blocks involved in synthesis and elimination as well.

So we eat food, and we digest it. The teeny tiny digested byproducts of the food—the teeny tiny amount of glucose from carbohydrates, amino acids from proteins, fatty acids from fats, vitamins and minerals—make it into the blood, circulate to the liver, and then on to all the cells of the body. All three byproducts, along with help from vitamins and minerals, can be "burned" as fuel to produce energy, can be biochemically transformed to produce cells, and thus, body structures; or, they can be part of the metabolic waste removal process.

In energy metabolism, glucose is like jet fuel: it burns "hot" through a process called "oxidation," and it combines with the oxygen we breathe. Glucose is the preferred fuel for high energy demand organs such as the brain,[17.1] as well as for many kinds of "fight-or-flight" needs because it provides quick and intense energy for rapid-fire metabolism. There is more to oxidation than just glucose. You may already know that excessive oxidation can be harmful to the body, which is why you hear so much about antioxidants. Because glucose is so quick to "oxidize," it is a less desirable molecule for ordinary day-to-day energy metabolism. Fats and amino acids are the more standard fuels and are preferable for maintaining daily energy needs; for example, for the ordinary needs of the heart and skeletal muscles as well as so many of the organs in our bodies. However, our brain in general, and when under increased demand, our heart and skeletal muscles,[17.1] do require glucose as their primary fuel.

Because of the potential for excessive oxidation, we have an exquisite system that carefully regulates glucose levels in the blood. At the core of this system is a hormone named insulin. Our body strongly monitors and adjusts the amount of glucose available in the blood at each moment: not too little and not too much. Our bodies also readily convert most surplus glucose into safer, slower-to-oxidize fats, such as triglycerides.

Our physiology aggressively prevents excesses of glucose in the blood by that significant insulin protective mechanism. Insulin reduces excessive blood glucose levels by causing the glucose to move out of the blood and into the cells (Figure 17a, next page). Insulin also encourages energy storage. Thus, interestingly, insulin also causes fats that are in the blood to move into and be stored in the cells.

The process of glucose regulation begins with digestion. Again, when a meal contains carbohydrates, these carbohydrates are digested and are broken down into glucose molecules. As soon as glucose is absorbed from the intestine,

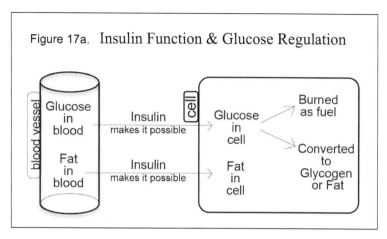

Figure 17a. Insulin Function & Glucose Regulation

it is transported into the blood of the portal vein (a blood vessel that goes from the intestine directly to the liver). The glucose level in the blood in this portal vein then rises (Figure 17b), and sensors detect the presence of this newly arrived glucose. If there is abundant glucose, that portal vein glucose level will rise above a threshold's upper limit. The sensors in the portal vein then call for the release of insulin. As a result of insulin action, much of the glucose from a meal is

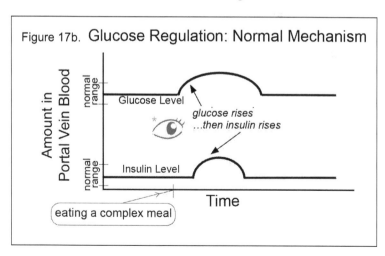

Figure 17b. Glucose Regulation: Normal Mechanism

 *The "eye" in this figure and those that follow represents a good place to begin your inspection of these drawings.*

immediately taken up by the liver cells. When that occurs, the portal vein blood glucose level falls below the upper limit of the optimal range, thereby terminating the need for and the secretion of insulin. Again, insulin facilitates the transport of glucose out of the blood and into the cells. Figure 17b on the preceding page shows what happens when a food has a slow and gradual digestion and absorption rate: this example depicts the process with a complex rather than a simple meal to digest and assimilate. Note that the glucose rise is gradual, as digestion is gradual. The insulin response is likewise gradual, and as the insulin rises, the glucose is moved out of the blood and into the cells. The blood glucose level then gradually falls, thus reducing the need for insulin, which then also gradually declines.

There is no immediate metabolic need for all of the glucose that would be available from any meal that contains *excessive* carbohydrates. Also, we wouldn't want excessive, easy-to-oxidize glucose "floating" about with no immediate purpose. Therefore, again, much of this glucose is taken up by and processed in the liver. In the liver, it is converted into molecules that can be stored well in the cells, such as "glycogen" (a reusable form of carbohydrate), or as a simple fat such as "triglycerides" (Figure 17c, next page).

Important characteristics of and facts related to these conversions include:

- The brain cells[17.1] almost exclusively burn glucose. All other body cells can burn either glucose, triglycerides and fatty acids, and/or amino acids. When bursts of energy are needed, organs such as active muscles or the heart, for example, can also utilize glucose.
- Glycogen can be converted back to glucose.

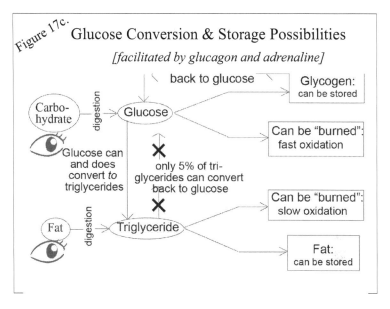

Figure 17c. **Glucose Conversion & Storage Possibilities**

*[facilitated by glucagon and adrenaline]*

- Triglycerides, as mentioned, can be distributed to and enter the cells, and can be "burned" as fuel or *stored as fat. Ooops.*

- Triglycerides, once produced *from glucose* (or fat), mostly *cannot be converted back into* glucose. Only the "glycerol" part of triglycerides can be converted back into glucose (glycerol is 5% of a triglyceride).

Again, fats are slower and relatively "quiet" in their oxidation. Thus, they can be a preferable molecule to burn. Fats also store easily—and abundantly, if necessary.

Our bodies store reserves of fuel so that they can be available for the times in the day (or our lives) when we are more active, and/or we are not eating or digesting. Glycogen is stored in the liver and the muscles, though not in large quantities. It has merit as a storage form as it can easily be converted into glucose to be used as an immediate high energy source. Fat is burned or stored, depending on the needs generated by basic living and physical activity. Fat is wonderful; it is only the *excessive* storage of fat that sooner or later in our lives, for so many of us, becomes a concern. Remember that one source of fat production can be from glucose, and glucose is the base of all carbohydrates!

Again, most but not all of our cells can burn either glucose and/or simple fats such as triglycerides to produce energy.[17.1] Triglycerides, although they are often derived from glucose, only 5% (the "glycerol" part of them) can be converted back into glucose. Thus, is not possible for your body to extract a significant amount of glucose from stored fat. Although it can pull that fat back into service as direct fat fuel for many cells, most of that fat (95%) cannot be converted back into glucose.

### Hypoglycemia and Adrenaline

When you don't listen to the words of your mother, and you skip your breakfast or other meals, your body will gradually use the glucose in your blood, causing it to decline below an acceptable level. Low blood glucose ("hypoglycemia") is intolerable for the body because, once again, many crucial cells, those in the brain, for example, need to create their energy from glucose. As your blood glucose levels begin to run low, mechanisms to restore your levels back to normal will come into play. One primary restoration mechanism is the sensation of *hunger* to motivate you to go forth and eat food. If you do not eat, another primary mechanism is to tap into glycogen reserves and convert glycogen into glucose. This conversion is facilitated by the hormones epinephrine (adrenaline) and glucagon (Figure 17c, page 225). Therefore, when you are hungry, you secrete adrenaline for assistance.

This can become mightily inconvenient if the low blood glucose, the hypoglycemia, occurs in the middle of the night while you are sleeping. That little jolt of protective adrenaline may also wake you up. No problem. Perhaps you'll go eat a snack. This isn't a problem for 20-year-olds; they seem to metabolize the adrenaline quite quickly so that they will fall back to sleep easily. However, at the 50,000-mile mark of menopause, for one thing, hypoglycemia is only one cause of nocturnal adrenaline: a nocturnal hot flash is also accompanied by adrenaline output. Also, women of menopausal age seem to have a slower biochemical degradation processing rate. So, whether your adrenaline came from middle-of-the-night hypoglycemia, from a hot flash, or from both, and whatever the biochemistry, you may find yourself staying awake awhile until the adrenaline is fully broken down and eliminated. Since adrenaline is quite energizing, you might even have quite an active, "racing" mind.

This is but one of the possible causes for sleep challenges in menopause. Low progesterone alone can do it, among others.

*Gluconeogenesis: Generating Glucose from Muscle Breakdown*

When glycogen reserves are too low, the body may resort to yet another mechanism to supply glucose. A type of hormone known as a "glucocorticoid" is secreted to stimulate the breakdown and conversion of protein into glucose in a process called "gluconeogenesis" (Figure 17d, next page).

The principle source of the protein that is utilized for this conversion to glucose is your muscles. Yikes! If you are starving or seriously calorie deprived, and your body is in need of glucose, you could eventually be breaking down your own muscles. Ooof! You may have thought that a too-

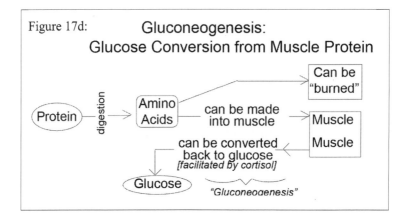

Figure 17d:
**Gluconeogenesis:**
**Glucose Conversion from Muscle Protein**

low calorie diet would help you lose fat but, in reality, you could be losing muscle! Whoa!

And, by the way, the principle glucocorticoid called upon to initiate gluconeogenesis is a stress hormone called cortisol! By missing meals, together with other dietary indiscretions that soon will be described, you can put a strain upon and "tire out" your cortisol/adrenal mechanisms, leading to "fatigue" of your adrenal glands. You can even adversely affect your immune system with the excess cortisol! Plus, you can increase insulin resistance.

*Glucose Regulation: Not Eating and Not Responding to Hunger*

Let's focus on this missed breakfast phenomenon in detail. Recall that when you haven't eaten for a length of time, your blood glucose level will start to fall, as illustrated in Figure 17e on the next page. When it falls beneath an acceptable threshold, you will get hungry. If you do not eat, the next step may be that glucose is mobilized from stored glycogen, and eventually, your blood glucose will be returned to acceptable levels. If the food deprivation goes on for too

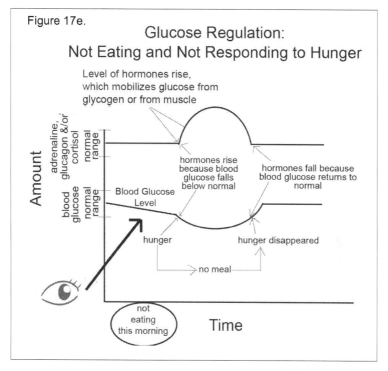

Figure 17e.

## Glucose Regulation:
## Not Eating and Not Responding to Hunger

Level of hormones rise, which mobilizes glucose from glycogen or from muscle

Amount

adrenaline, glucagon &/or cortisol — normal range

blood glucose — normal range

Blood Glucose Level

hormones rise because blood glucose falls below normal

hormones fall because blood glucose returns to normal

hunger

hunger disappeared

no meal

not eating this morning

Time

long, along with fat storage meeting some but not all energy needs, you can eventually break down muscle and turn it into glucose, again, through the process of gluconeogenesis that is facilitated by cortisol. Yes, you will break down and utilize fat for energy. However, the body still needs glucose, and if it cannot get it from food or glycogen, it will generate it from protein by gluconeogenesis.

Have you ever been hungry, not eaten, and nevertheless noticed after a while that your hunger had disappeared? Long before I became a doctor, I noticed and was mystified by this curious phenomenon. I'd be super-hungry, but not eat, and then, a little while later I'd notice that I was no longer hungry! That sensation of hunger occurred because our brains detected low blood glucose and gave us a strong signal to go out foraging for food. The hunger disappeared because our bodies were secreting adrenaline, glucagon, and cortisol, and accessing stored fuel from glycogen. And, if need be because glycogen reserves are low, our bodies will break down muscle to raise blood glucose. Once again, it is the cortisol that initiates gluconeogenesis. Also, these hormones are appetite suppressive in their own right!

*Glucose Regulation: The Challenge of Simple Carbohydrates*

One of the most challenging issues for the glucose regulating mechanism is the eating of simple carbohydrates. You know carbohydrates are *"simple"* if they are *sweet.* In Figure 17f, we see what happens when a person eats or drinks something sweet, such as a can of soda pop, which typically contains several teaspoons of sugar. This stuff is so "simple"

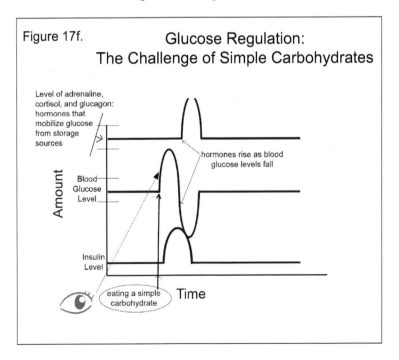

Figure 17f. **Glucose Regulation: The Challenge of Simple Carbohydrates**

that almost no digestion is required; the sugar is absorbed immediately, and blood glucose levels rise very quickly and all at once. Glucose levels, in this case, go much higher than with complex carbohydrates that digest and assimilate more slowly over time (Figure 17b, page 223 and repeated below). This rapid rise in glucose (Figure 17f, preceding page) fools the insulin response. At levels this high, your body thinks that you must have eaten a very large meal, with more carbohydrates to come. (Genetically, our bodies haven't quite acclimated to the fact that carbohydrates can be anything but com-

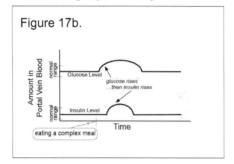

Figure 17b.

plex.) So, you secrete a large amount of insulin. Well, in this case, there was no substantial, slower-to-digest complex carbohydrate following the sugar in that can of soda. Your body overestimates. Thus, the excess insulin causes a plummet in your glucose level. This plummet—known as "hypoglycemia"— is unacceptable for the body and, once again, adrenaline, glucagon, and glucocorticoids are called to rescue. This pattern of eating simple carbohydrates (mainly sweets) leads to more problems for human beings than almost any other dietary indiscretion!

## *Excess Carbohydrates, Stress, and Insulin Resistance*

Do adrenaline and cortisol sound familiar? They are the main hormonal first-responders in times of stress. Stress, of course, has increased metabolic needs, and these stress hormones supply the extra fuel the body requires at these times of "fight-or-flight."

Excessive adrenaline and cortisol lead to biological in-sulin resistance (!), which is harmful. In this phenomenon, insulin just does not work as well. To overcome this resis-tance, higher than normal insulin levels are now required to get the desired insulin effect. Another cause of insulin resistance is the long-term overstimulation of insulin from the excessive intake of carbohydrates. As insulin resistance develops, glucose, triglyceride, and cholesterol have more difficulty entering the cells to be utilized as fuel. As a re-sult, these levels rise in the blood. If you see high levels of cholesterol and triglycerides on your blood test results, they are commonly caused by insulin resistance provoked by excessive carbohydrate intake.

## *Weight Loss and the Fat Myth*

The common strategy to lose weight by reducing fats can pose a problem. Fats have acquired such a flawed and not totally deserved reputation. In general, the American diet, compared to years ago, has fewer fats, a lot of the time by per-sonal choice. As a consequence of the reduction of fats and as a way to make up for the lost calories, the amount of car-bohydrates has increased in the diet! Many of the excessive carbohydrates will be converted into fat, and much of *that* fat will be stored. Plus, if you eat excessive carbohydrates, you will need to generate more insulin, which will result in higher than optimal levels. Eventually, you will wear down your ability to produce adequate insulin in the same manner that hormone production is diminished because of long-term overuse of chronic stress. This, along with insulin resistance, eventually leads to unbeneficial elevations in blood glucose levels known as diabetes.

***Overeating simple carbohydrates
(mainly sweets, bread, pastries, and soft drinks)
leads to more problems for human beings
than almost any other dietary indiscretion!***

Of course, there are other factors. Again, stress raises adrenaline and cortisol levels, and these contribute to insulin resistance. Stimulants such as caffeine and nicotine have the same effect. Look at the possibilities: overeating carbohydrates, skipping meals, and stress all lead to elevated insulin, elevated cortisol and adrenaline, and insulin resistance. When you are no longer young (but still eating as if you were) and if you become less physically active, the fat deposition increases. Thus, you diet, and you reduce the fat content in your meals because you are afraid of fat. When you reduce the fat, which represents a significant reduction in calories, you become hungry and compensate by increasing your carbohydrate intake! But you want to lose weight, so you think that you need to reduce your calories. However, your brain et al. needs glucose, so adrenaline and cortisol are secreted, and you even run the risk of converting your muscles into glucose. Insulin levels rise. Yet, you continue to eat carbohydrates. You store more fat!

***Look at the possibilities:
overeating carbohydrates, skipping meals,
and stress all lead to elevated insulin, cortisol
and adrenaline, as well as to insulin resistance.***

Because of estrogen, women tend to deposit fat in their hips and thighs. Because of testosterone, men tend to accumulate it in their abdomen. When women start depositing fat into their abdomen, we know that insulin resistance has progressed, and triglyceride blood levels have increased. Sooner or later, insulin increases and cholesterol is dumped into the cells. Plus, you break down your muscle to yield amino acids for gluconeogenesis! Get the picture?

> *If this sounds utterly circular and hopelessly entwangled, it is. And all of these errors drive you to increased weight gain.*

*Calories, Metabolism, Appetite, and Nutrient Rich Foods*

Any discussion of weight gain would be incomplete without mention of the subjects of reducing excessive calories, choosing nutrient-rich foods, and addressing an excessive appetite! Calorie strategy for weight loss requires planning with significant technical skill and detail. Following a diet that is based upon a calorie reduction plan and maintaining weight loss is a challenge and an art, and it also requires substantial willpower. It is suspect for physiologic reasons and, most often, fails in the long run. As effective as you would think carefully designed caloric restriction might be, it can become very difficult to execute. All of the information I have discussed must be taken into consideration:

- One significant issue is that if you reduce your calorie intake, you increase your hunger! Yikes. Often, this is what marks the end for serious calorie counters: hunger is one major and difficult barrier to overcome for long-term success.

- Also, if you decide to lower calories by skipping breakfast, for example, you can call adrenaline and cortisol into action to raise your falling blood glucose level. However, you will only fool yourself. These stress hormones will raise blood glucose and suppress appetite. However, they will also increase resistance to insulin. By lunch, the carbohydrates that you eat will call for insulin in the face of that increased resistance, so higher levels of insulin will be required. This will accelerate fat creation and deposition!

- Long-term calorie deprivation just doesn't work for yet another reason. Your body will slow down metabolism as it realizes that you are not providing sufficient food for all of its many needs. You will not "burn off the pounds" you had hoped for because your "burn" biochemistry (metabolism) has been ratcheted down.

- Use of non-organic food. Agribusiness food contains a significantly reduced nutrient content. You can eat a meal that has adequate calories but contains only a reduced percentage of the vitamin and mineral content it should have. You try to leave the table, yet you have cravings for the vitamins and minerals that were deficient. These cravings translate into the desire to graze through more food (thus more calories!) to obtain the missing nutrients.

## Neurotransmitters and Appetite

Curbing appetite can be part of the equation for weight reduction. Sometimes, an excessive appetite is associated with diminished neurotransmitters. This is a topic unto itself. To further your understanding:

- Principle neurotransmitters can diminish over time by the same mechanism in which a dysfunctional response to stress can cause the overproduction and then ultimate fatigue of the glands that produce hormones.

- Serotonin is a common neurotransmitter that is so often depleted in adults. We do know that replenishing it in some folks can reduce appetite. My preferred way to do so is by supplementing with the amino acid 5-hydroxytryptophan, together with vitamin and mineral cofactors. This has known appetite-suppressing capabilities:[17.2] it can calm down an excessive appetite! As with any nutritional supplement (or hormone or pharmaceutical medication), individuality matters, so a trial is warranted. It does not guarantee success, in this case appetite reduction, yet oh my, when it works, it is a major blessing. Although pharmaceutical medications ("SSRIs") artificially increase serotonin levels, they commonly have weight gain associated with them (for reasons that are not entirely clear).

- It is interesting to recall that years ago there was a very popular and effective appetite suppressant, Dexedrine, known back in the day as the "diet pill." It is an amphetamine, which is an artificial and long-acting adrenaline. It worked because adrenaline, besides being a major hormone of adrenal origin, is a principle neurotransmitter. It turns out that if you are lower in adrenaline, you can experience an increased appetite. Those who took Dexadrine had a major decrease in appetite! (I won't go into the intense downsides of this amphetamine, nor those of "fen-phen." The latter was removed from the market and banned because of *serious* side effects!)

- Adrenaline and noradrenaline levels can be directly supported by taking the nutritional precursors to them in supplement form. These are based on the amino acid precursor, L-Tyrosine.[17.3]

• Neurotransmitter levels can be tested. I have been using a commercial laboratory for testing neurotransmitters in my patients for many years. I so often see neurotransmitter test results that correlate well with the patient's clinical situation. It is so common to see depleted serotonin as well as depleted catecholamines (adrenaline and noradrenaline). A practitioner who is knowledgeable in this field can assist you with neurotransmitter restoration. When repletion is addressed skillfully, with targeted nutritional supplementation, improvements can and do occur! Improvements can include successful appetite suppression as well as mood restorations. Many who find that these supplements work for them—actually, beyond theory—benefit from and appreciate them greatly!

There is a myriad of additional factors that affect our appetite for food. Here are a few more:

• Self "medicating." Are you really hungry or eating out of habit and boredom to give yourself a simple pleasure when you are feeling "low," or as a substitute for hunger for other things in life?

• Repression. Are you using food to "quiet down" uncomfortable emotions?

### More about Hormones and Metabolic Burn Rate

As a final consideration, let's test your strength and endurance by tying all of this in with hormones! As I have mentioned before, technically, metabolism is dependent upon many factors including thyroid hormone function. Thyroid function is a major determiner of the metabolic rate of burn: low thyroid, then low energy metabolism... and a tired patient. It is hard to lose weight when you are functionally low in thyroid hormone. Proper thyroid hormone function can itself be dependent upon adequate progesterone levels. Once again, we see the importance of hormones in general, and of progesterone, the latter of which all but disappears in menopause, even in perimenopause, and sometimes as early as the mid-thirties.

Identifying and treating functional thyroid lowness (a gland that is just not putting out quite enough hormones as it is "fatigued") often takes a medical professional with special training in this phenomenon: usually a holistic, functional, or complementary physician. Standard thyroid blood tests will not necessarily identify this condition. For completeness, I recommend a blood test that includes TSH, free T4, free T3, and reverse T3. A TSH > 2 is suspect.

Excessive insulin affects hormones. It can cause an increase in androgens. This increase can interfere with ovulation in young women. Egg development depends on the binding of estradiol to the cell surface of the maturing ovum. Increased androgens can interfere with that binding. Maturation can be blocked as well as the needed luteinizing hormone (LH) surge, thereby interfering with ovulation. The absence of ovulation results in greatly diminished progesterone. Diminishing insulin through insulin-lowering (carbohydrate lowering) choices can often restore normal periods in a younger woman!

Birth control pills have an artificial progesterone in them ("progestins") that behave more like testosterone than progesterone. Taking birth control pills to restore or regulate periods during menopause can be plenty problematic for weight.

Estrogens enhance insulin sensitivity. Diminished estrogen is accompanied by diminished insulin sensitivity, for instance, insulin resistance. Follow that thought, as it ties into menopause and weight gain.

Estrogen is an excellent stress hormone. It's not "front of the pack" like adrenaline or cortisol, yet when stressed, a woman's body will contribute estrogens to the fight-or-flight hormonal mix. In a young, stressed woman, estrogens shunted down the stress pathway will not be available to support the formation of the endometrial lining. This is why many young women, stressed by life or intense athletics, miss or lose their periods. As estrogens decline in menopause, and if there is stress, the body will often need to increase the amount of cortisol in the "mix" to compensate further for the absence of estrogens. Increased cortisol raises blood glucose and enhances insulin resistance. Round and round we go.

## Digestion and Assimilation of Food

The food we purchase and prepare goes into our mouth. Then what? Well, some foods are super easy to digest and assimilate into our bodies, and others are not so easy. A peach requires so little effort or saliva, internal stomach acids, and pancreatic enzymes to digest. Chicken, on the other hand, requires some highly-sophisticated processes and digestive juices! It all begins with chewing! It's a physics principle: the "surface area to solvent ratio." If you put a one-half-square-inch bite of chicken into your mouth, there are a range of possibilities between:

- you swallow it whole, or
- you chew it so thoroughly that it turns to liquid in your mouth.

Which works better for digestion? You bet. Chewing very thoroughly breaks foods down into teeny tiny particles that dissolve so much better when they are subjected to the stomach's hydrochloric acid and pancreatic digestive enzymes. As we age, the hydrochloric acid and pancreatic enzymes diminish, and the ability to digest declines! How does this affect our weight? When you eat any meal, and you have a compromised digestion, what *does* digest are the easy foodstuffs: the carbohydrates. What doesn't digest as well, and thus partially winds up in our bodies, and ultimately, partially winds up in the toilet, are proteins and fats. Yet proteins and fats are essential; if we do not assimilate sufficient amino acids from proteins and essential fatty acids from fats, our bodies remain hungry for what we didn't get. Then comes the message to graze through more food, thus causing you to ingest more calories, in hopes of acquiring the missing nutrients.

The remedies include:

- Chew, chew, chew, chew, and chew.

- Supplement digestive enzymes and, if tolerated, betaine hydrochloride (see www.iwonderdoctor/digestion).

- And oh, by the way, eat at a nice slow pace. For one thing, it takes at least 20 minutes into a meal for enough of the digested food to enter into your body and be registered sufficiently for you to get the message that you are satisfied. If you are bolting down a meal in 10 minutes, you may eat quite a bit more than you need as you may not have received the message that you are satisfied!

Please view Figure 17g ( a summary chart of the outcome of carbohydrates, proteins, and fats) on the following page. I do acknowledge that this chapter can inspire one to howl at the moon!

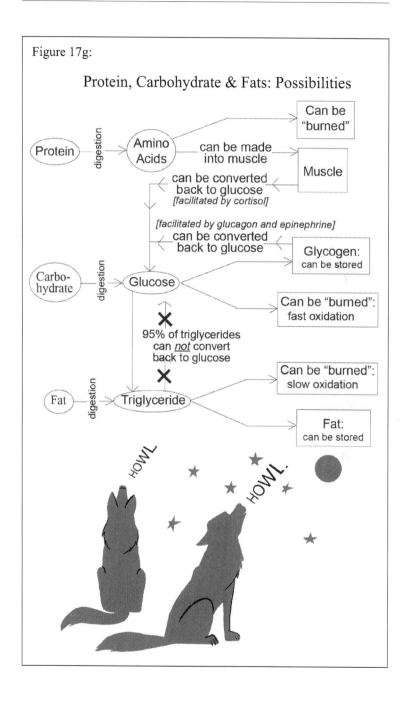

Figure 17g:

Protein, Carbohydrate & Fats: Possibilities

*Summary of Weight Issues*

Thus, we see that many factors can influence a woman's body weight during the perimenopausal and menopausal years. Once again, for your review, these include the following:

- Excessive intake of carbohydrates, especially simple carbohydrates (the worst case: almost anything sweet. Also, breads, pastries, soda pop, etc.).

- Diminished ability to physiologically manage carbohydrates (glucose/insulin regulating issues).

- Increased insulin resistance caused by excessive carbohydrates, adrenaline, cortisol, glucagon, and by diminished estrogens.

- Diminished hormones such as estrogen, progesterone, and soon, if not already, testosterone and DHEA, as well as the distinct possibility of lowish thyroid levels.

- Decreasing metabolic rate of caloric "burn" caused by a variety of reasons, including hormonal decline as well as significant calorie restriction.

- An exaggerated response to stress that triggers excessive stress hormones, thus blood glucose elevations and insulin resistance.

- Insufficient physical activity.

- Reduced neurotransmitter levels, especially serotonin and the catecholamines (e.g., adrenaline and noradrenaline), leading to an excessive appetite.

- Nutrient depletion in non-organic foods, resulting in additional hunger for missing nutrients. Consequently, we graze through and consume additional food, thus calories, in a quest to meet minimum nutritional needs—especially those of depleted minerals and vitamins.

- Eating to "quiet" your uncomfortable emotions or to fill up your hunger for what you feel is missing.

- Reduced ability to digest and assimilate what we eat, causing an increased appetite to make up for what we didn't digest or absorb.

- Other causes, such as an intestinal yeast infection.

*Summary of Weight Loss Strategies*

A simplified approach to the complex subject of weight in menopausal women looks like this:

- Exercise, exercise, and exercise. Not stressfully, not to excess. And by the way, be sure to exercise.

- If you are eating an excessive amount of carbohydrates and sweets, reduce this amount.

- Eat *organic* food as much as possible so that the food you do eat has the maximum amount of nutrients available and does not leave you hungry, causing you to graze through more calories to chase after missing nutrients.

- Chew, chew, chew. Consider taking digestive enzymes and betaine hydrochloride to assist digestion.

- Eat slowly enough so that your brain will actually have time to register that you are satisfied.

- Eat whole foods and minimize processed foods.

- Make the effort to minimize the release of excessive insulin by:

- ○ Reducing carbohydrate intake.

- ○ Reducing excessive and inappropriate responses to stress.

- ○ Reducing stimulants such as caffeine and nicotine.

- ○ Increasing exercise if you're not "up to speed."

- Acquire additional information to do well with stress. Stress is likely to be encountered; however, it isn't the stress that is the problem. Make an effort to identify and heal the "elephant in the room," which, bottom line, are any uncomfortable emotions and thoughts that occur within us and are ours to heal. This is our leverage and one pillar of our spiritual growth (see www.iwonderdoctor.com/anxiety-and-depresssion).

- Seek professional assistance in evaluating, replenishing, and balancing all hormones that need it.

- Address neurotransmitters to normalize appetite.

- Eliminate hunger! If you get hungry, it actually means your blood glucose has fallen too low and triggered that super-strong feeling! Eat before that hunger occurs so that you do not provoke, besides the hunger, the adrenaline and cortisol rescue response!

- Eat small meals and snacks throughout the day. It's preemptive blood glucose management, and smaller meals are much easier to digest.

- Identify the foods that you react to (food "allergies") and eliminate them. A nutritionist or nutritionally-oriented health professional can assist you with this process.

- Take nutritional supplements: a high-quality multiple vitamin and mineral, omega-3 fish oil, vitamin C, and others. By doing so, you will meet the augmented nutritional needs caused by certain stresses in your life that you may not yet have acquired the skills to do well with. Supplements will also provide many of the nutrients that may not be present in our food because of farming methods or distance and time from farm to table.

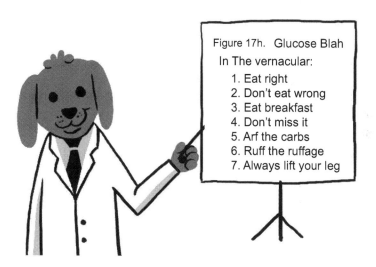

Figure 17h. Glucose Blah

In The vernacular:

1. Eat right
2. Don't eat wrong
3. Eat breakfast
4. Don't miss it
5. Arf the carbs
6. Ruff the ruffage
7. Always lift your leg

Chapter Eighteen

# In Praise and Honor of the Bladder: Squeeze!

There are so many women who face challenges somewhere along the way related to peeing! Likewise, there are many elderly women who are incontinent and are wearing seriously padded underwear. How did this come about?

I was speaking recently with my colleague Nancy, a seasoned veteran nurse practitioner who specializes in treating the elderly as well as in hormone replenishment. She was telling me about a woman who gave birth to four 10 lb. babies. We both knew what that could mean with regard to stress on her pelvic muscular support and her bladder. Add to this the changes of untreated menopause: vaginal atrophy with subsequent vulnerability and proneness to irritability of the urethral meatus (where the tube coming from the bladder empties into the vagina), and the crucial last straw is the weakening of the amazing muscular support that "holds up" the bladder, the levator ani. This weakening occurs primarily because of the loss of androgens(!) and also because of neglect.

The remedy? Once again, an ounce of prevention is worth a ton of cure:

- "Kegels:" Dr. Kegel was an American gynecologist who studied the support of the pelvic floor and popularized the crucial importance of exercising its wonderful main muscle, the levator ani. Here's how you do it:

  ○ Focus your attention on squeezing your anus as tight as you can—and then relaxing it. This is the same muscle that supports your bladder, uterus, and vagina. It's the muscle you use to try to "hold your pee."

o Of the many rituals women have invented to remember to do these exercises, Nancy[18.1] told me about her favorite advice to all of her patients: write a reminder on an index card and place it above your toilet paper roll. My favorite reminder word is "squeeze!" Squeeze 10 times every time you sit on the toilet. Add that up!

o I am a devotee of the YMCA. Two-thirds of the exercisers there on any given day are women who wouldn't dream of missing their exercise! Just add the big squeeze to your daily regimen as early in life as you possibly can. You'll be forever grateful!

• Bio-identical hormone treatment!

o The health of your vagina depends on estrogens! It will atrophy without them. The urethral meatus is part of the vaginal tissue where it opens into the vagina. That point of entry is very vulnerable to atrophy and can become easily irritated and, thus, is a source of recurrent bladder infections.

o Androgens, androgens, androgens: testosterone and DHEA. By the time of menopause, most women will already be experiencing a significant decline in androgens because of their excessive response to stress over the years. Some may not. Your health professional can help you sort that out. In my experience, *all* women, by the time they reach 2 to 5 years into menopause, will have serious androgen depletion. The health and strength of the muscles throughout your body depend on androgens. When you see the elderly women in walkers and wheelchairs, it is most often because of sarcopenia (the loss of muscle mass and strength). Now picture your beloved levator ani.

- It's never too late:
  - It's never too late for hormones.
  - It's never too late for the gym.
  - It's never too late for the big squeeze!

Nancy told me that the patient with the four 10 lb. babies developed one recurrent bladder infection after another in her eighties, all of which ceased when Nancy started her on the MM-Elder hormone formulation (see Chapter 13).

Chapter Nineteen

## ... In Closing ...

I hope that this book has been helpful to you. The beginning of this journey is often daunting —reading about it certainly is—but it gets easier, I assure you. So many women have been successful, both in dealing with the changes brought on by this new phase of life and also with the steps before them to best thrive in it.

The good news is that the majority of women figure it out. It can be no big deal, indeed, rather easy, or it can seem complex and overwhelming. And it can be wonderful in its own way, too. Menopause occurs at a true time of change: it is a genuine portal into a new life stage, every bit as important as the several life stages that preceded it.

Certainly, the "hormonology" has a complexity to it, but once the adjustments and possible readjustments to your protocol achieve success, the gratitude sets in.

Menopause, for so many of my patients, is a time of "return," a shift away from so much involvement in the world of "10,000 things." It is a journey to deeper places, often described to me as an "uncovering" of new ease, wisdom, and peace, "a coming home," a "spiritual awakening." This can be the most rewarding part of all!

I wish you all so well,

Dr. R

# Acknowledgments

This book exists because of the support and collaboration of many people.

Again, the foundation of so much that I understand of menopause comes from working with my many women patients over the years. Their biggest gift has always been who they are. Yet, it has been the heat of many a flash and the sorting out of their individual details that has kept my feet to the fire to get this one right.

I thank the pioneers in the field of bio-identical female hormone medicine, including Jonathan Wright M.D., John Lee M.D., and Eugene Shippen M.D., among many others, who have made such a difference. Thank you to Jonathan and Gene for your special friendships.

Gratitude to the laboratories and compounding pharmacists, so many of whom stand out for their knowledge, support, and the quality of their work. Among them, special thanks to my long-time colleagues and friends, Frank Nordt Ph.D. of Rhein Consulting Laboratories and Tom White R.Ph., Ph.C. of TW Wellness. And thank you to the many physicians and scientists behind the countless studies in our medical literature.

Beyond menopause, I'm grateful to Jeff Bland Ph.D. who has contributed so extensively to my knowledge, and that of so many.

Catherine Logan, Brett Jacques N.D., Betsy Cole, and David Perlmutter M.D., thanks for your support in the initial phases of this project. Thank you to the many people who are and have been caring and supportive of me and this work over the years: Lyn Marsh Ph.D., Fran Lankford, Gina James, Kathy McDonald, Eisa Lindner, Donna Wolfe ARNP, and Mary Hickland.

Again, to Shea Lindner, thank you for your hours and hours, ease, strength, brilliance, grace, and humor in the early editions. Sheree Mikulec, thank you for your impeccable editing, enthusiasm, caring, kindness, precision, and endless efforts. Gennie Fassanella, your artistic renderings of Shea and my cartoons bring a delightful smile when I see them.

Again, with much gratitude, and the best to you all.

Also, and most personally of all,

My mother and father, Paula and Marty, for their love and space;

Paula and Mary for inspiring MM-Elder;

Jen, my daughter;

Joshua, my amazing son and extraordinary partner.
The Menopause Method exists because you and I decided to do all of this together;

My beloved Kim, for the gift of who you are, for your love, and for being able to care about and love you;

Maya and Mali, in a time so long ago and far away...

# Illustration Credits

Caleb Bish: pages 123, 305

Gennie Fasanella (gefasanella@gmail.com): pages 37, 41, 51, 53, 71, 83, 88, 90, 91, 92, 93, 96, 112, 113, 125, 132, 138, 154, 159, 162, 163, 208, 217, 241, 244

Donna Hicks: page 123

Michael Lam M.D: page 14
http://www.drlam.com/articles/estrogen_dominance.asp

Shea Lindner conceived and illustrated original illustrations in editions 1–5: pages 25, 37, 41, 51, 53, 71, 83, 88, 90, 91, 92, 93, 96, 112, 113, 125, 132, 138, 154, 159, 162, 163, 208, 217, 241, 244

Joshua Rosensweet: pages 49, 50, 76, 79, 80, 81, 82, 84, 119, 120, 122, 123, 124, 129, 130, 304

Daved Rosensweet, M.D.: pages 76, 79, 80, 81, 82, 84, 119, 120, 122, 123, 124, 129, 130, 304
Conceived and illustrated all graphs except page 14
Conceived original illustrations in editions 1–5: pages 25, 37, 41, 51, 53, 71, 83, 88, 90, 91, 92, 93, 96, 112, 113, 125, 132, 138, 154, 159, 162, 163, 208, 217, 241, 244

Sarfraz Sama (qnonym@gmail.com): pages 49, 50

Parin Sorathiya: pages 49, 50

# References from Chapters

**Chapter Two:**
**Menopause: An Introduction**
2.1   Michael Lam, M.D.
      https://www.drlam.com/articles/estrogen_dominance.asp

**Chapter Three:**
**Risk and Benefits**
3.1   See Appendix B, references 10 and 11
      10. Women's Health Initiative (WHI) and the Issues
          Related to It
      11. Hormone Treatment and Breast Cancer Risk
          (Regarding the two arms of the WHI study)
3.2   See Appendix B, references 8 and 9
      8.  Breast Cancer Risk: Mainstream View
      9.  Estrogen: Breast Cancer, Trophic or Initiator?
3.3   See Appendix B, references 21, 22, and 23
      21. Holtorf's Review: Are Bio-identical Hormones
          Safer or More Efficacious?
      22. Transdermal Hormone Rx & Risk
      23. Unequal risks for breast cancer associated with
          different hormone replacement therapies.
3.4   See Appendix B, references 1 and 2
      1.  Estrogen and Coronary Artery Disease
      2.  Cardiovascular and cancer safety of
          testosterone in women.
3.5   See Appendix B, references 3, 4, 5, 6, and 7
      3.  Estrogen and Memory
      4.  Estrogen and Alzheimer's Disease
      5.  HRT and Weight Gain
      6.  Estrogen Dose Levels and Bone Density

**(Chapter Three, continued)**

    7. Estrogen Neuroprotection and the Critical Period Hypothesis: [Review article]

3.6  See Appendix B, references 21, 22, and 23

    21. Holtorf's Review: Are Bio-identical Hormones Safer or More Efficacious?

    22. Transdermal Hormone Rx & Risk

    23. Unequal risks for breast cancer associated with different hormone replacement therapies.

3.7  See Appendix B, reference 32

    32. Oral Estradiol: Increased Hormone & Metabolite Issues

**Chapter Six:**
**Progesterone**

6.1  John Lee, M.D.
https://www.johnleemd.com/enlarged-uterus-fi-broids-hormone-imbalance-estrogen-dominance.html

6.2  Christiane Northrup, M.D.
http://www.drnorthrup.com/fibroids/

6.3  Jason D. Wright, MD, et al. Nationwide Trends in the Performance of Inpatient Hysterectomy in the United States.
*Obstet Gynecol.* 2013 Aug; 122(2 0 1): 233–241.

**Chapter Seven:**
**Estrogens**

7.1  See Appendix B, references 79, 80, and 81

    79. Reduced Estriol Excretion in Patients with Breast Cancer Prior to Endocrine Therapy

    80. Reducing the Hormone Related Cancer Risk (Or cabbages, sex hormones and their metabolites)

81. Jonathan V. Wright M.D. Estriol: Its Weakness is Its Strength

7.2   See Appendix B, references 24 and 25

24. Breast Cancer Risk and the 2 Estrogen Receptors

25. Estriol Preferentially Binds to ERβ

7.3   Personal communication: Frank Nordt. Ph.D., of Rhein Consulting Laboratories

7.4   See Appendix B, references 28, 29, and 30

28. Are all estrogens created equal? A review of oral vs. transdermal therapy.

29. Oral Estrogen: Metabolite, Coagulation, and Other Issues

30. Coagulation Issues Matter

7.5   See Appendix B, reference 33

33. Transdermal vs Oral Estrogen: Another Resource

7.6   See Appendix B, references 29, 30, 77, and 78

29. Oral Estrogen: Metabolite, Coagulation, and Other Issues

30. Coagulation Issues Matter

77. Estrogen and Coagulation

78. Effects of oral and transdermal estrogen/pro-gesterone regimens on blood coagulation and fibrinolysis in postmenopausal women. A randomized controlled trial.

**Chapter Eight:**
**Hormone Dose Determination**

See Chart: Finding Your Optimal Dose of Estrogen by Titrating Between the Symptoms of Deficiency and Excess, page 326

**Chapter Nine:**
**Application Sites and Methods**
9.1 See Appendix B, references 74 and 82
74. Transdermal Transmission?
82. Are Transdermal Hormones Transmitted to Spouse and Others by Contact?
9.2 See Appendix B, reference 20
20. The Mortality Toll of Estrogen Avoidance: An Analysis of Excess Deaths Among Hysterecto-mized Women Aged 50 to 59 Years
9.3 See Appendix B, reference 52
52. Bio-identical Hormones: What's Fact and What's Fable?
9.4 See Appendix B, references 43, 44, 45, 46, and 47
43. Low Dose TD Carbopol Gel Improves HF + Vulvovaginal Atrophy
44. Transdemal estradiol gel for the treatment of symptomatic postmenopausal women.
45. Dose Levels & Bone Density
46. Dose Levels & Vaginal Atrophy (Patch)
47. Effects of Ultra-Low-Dose Transdermal Estradiol on Cognition and Health-Related Quality of Life
9.5 Go to the Institute for Functional Medicine for a referral to trained health professionals. Search for writings of Dale Bredesen, M.D., and Jeffrey Bland, Ph.D.
9.6 "Dermal fatigue" was first pointed out to me by Jonathan V. Wright, M.D.—one of his multitude of contributions to treatment with bio-identical hormones.
9.7 Estriol Vaginal Residual as Documented by Hormone Testing: My patient, F.G., applied estriol intravaginally. For the purposes of testing her by 24-hour urine col-

lection—because the urethral meatus empties into the distal vagina; thus, urine washes over the vaginal mucosa, which could possibly contain residual estriol—60 hours prior to testing, she stopped applying vaginal estriol. Nonetheless, the test results showed extremely high levels of estriol, indicating that estriol lingered in the vaginal mucosa much longer than we anticipated! This suggests that if women who are having intercourse are using vaginal estrogen, it could easily pass to their partner! F.G. was tested again months after having discontinued vaginal estriol. Her urine tested with normal expected levels of estriol.

**Chapter Ten:**
**Formulations: The Hormones, Carriers, and Dispensing Methods**

10.1  See Appendix B, references 36 and 37
    36. Carbopol ("Carbomer," etc.)
    37. Propylene Glycol Toxicity

10.2  Candace Newman (the "oil" lady)
    https://www.oilladyaromatherapy.com

10.3  *Explanation of "mgeeq"*
- Estradiol (E2) is the most potent estrogen.
- Estrone (E1) is 80% as strong as E2.
- Estriol is 12.5% as strong as E2.
- To assess the potency of a Bi-Est formula, in this case, 30 mg/ml 80:20 (80% E3, 20% E2), we do the following math. Since:
    - 20% of the formula is E2,
        - the E2 concentration equals 0.2 x 30 mg/ml = 6 mg/ml.
    - 80% is E3,
        - thus, 0.8 x 30 mg/ml = 24 mg/ml.
- As far as the potency goes however, if we assign a

**(Chapter Ten, continued)**

potency of 1 to E2, then the potency of E3 equals 0.125 x 24 mg/ml = 3 mg/ml.

- Thus, the total potency compared to the potency of pure estradiol equals 6 + 3 = 9 mgeeq.
- Therefore, 1 ml of Bi-Est 30 mg/ml 80:20 has a potency equivalent to 9 mg of estradiol, or, "9 mgeeq" (9 milligrams estradiol equivalency).
- Since there are 25 drops of Bi-Est in the organic oils formulation,
  - 1 drop contains 9 mgeeq/25 drops per ml = 0.36 mgeeq/drop.
- To fully understand this concept, I suggest doing the math. We round off and estimate that each drop of Bi-Est 30 mg/ml 80:20 has approximately 0.4 mgeeq, or to say it another way, each drop of this Bi-Est has a potency equivalent to 0.4 mg of estradiol.
- Enjoy the math... it's very useful clinically. In my practice, my satisfied menopausal patients, having titrated to what they consider optimal Bi-Est dosage sufficient to alleviate their estrogen deficiency symptoms, averages 1.7 mgeeq per day, divided into two dosages, morning and night (approximately 2 drops twice per day). My patients' dosage range from 0.8 to 2.6 mgeeq as there are variables in need, sensitivity, and absorption.

**Chapter Eleven:**
**Androgens**

See Chart: Finding Your Optimal Dose of Testosterone by Titrating Between the Symptoms of Deficiency and Excess, page 327

**Chapter Twelve:**
**Additional Details About Hormone Treatment**
12.1  See Appendix B, reference 52
52. Bio-identical Hormones: What's Fact and What's Fable?

**Chapter Thirteen:**
**Treating Elderly Women with Hormones**
13.1  See Appendix B, references 28, 29, 30, 77, and 78
28. Are all estrogens created equal? A review of oral vs transdermal therapy.
29. Oral Estrogen: Metabolite, Coagulation, and Other Issues
30. Coagulation Issues Matter
77. Estrogen and Coagulation
78. Effects of oral and transdermal estrogen/progesterone regimens on blood coagulation and fibrinolysis in postmenopausal women. A randomized controlled trial.
13.2  See Appendix A, illustrations of hormone test results

**Chapter Fourteen:**
**Patient Assessment: Initial and Ongoing**
14.1  See Appendix B, references 44, 45, 46, and 47
44. Transdermal estradiol gel for the treatment of symptomatic postmenopausal women.
45. Dose Levels & Bone Density
46. Dose Levels & Vaginal Atrophy (Patch)
47. Effects of Ultra-Low-Dose Transdermal Estradiol on Cognition and Health-Related Quality of Life
14.2  See Appendix B, references 3, 4, 7, and 47

    3. Estrogen and Memory

**(Chapter Fourteen, continued)**

    4. Estrogen and Alzheimer's Disease

    7. Estrogen Neuroprotection and the Critical Period Hypothesis: [Review article]

    47. Effects of Ultra-Low-Dose Transdermal Estradiol on Cognition and Health-Related Quality of Life

14.3 See Appendix B, reference 52

    52. Bio-identical Hormones: What's Fact and What's Fable?

**Chapter Fifteen:**
**Patient Assessment:**
**Fundamental Female Evaluations**

15.1 For further information regarding breast issues, you may like to read *Dressed to Kill: The Link Between Breast Cancer and Bras* by Sidney Ross Singer and Soma Grismaijer

15.2 See article by Dr. Joseph Mercola: Top Tips to Decrease Your Breast Cancer Risk http://articles.mercola.com/sites/articles/archive/2014/06/02/breast-cancer-prevention-strategies.aspx

15.3 Regarding sagging breasts: http://www.007b.com/sagging.php

15.4 Also, http://www.brafree.org

15.5 Alan Gaby, M.D., Editorial, rebuttals and responses regarding iodine http://www.townsendletter.com/July2006/iodine_gaby_0706.htm

15.6 See Appendix B, references 43, 44, 45, and 46

    43. Low Dose TD Carbopol Gel Improves HF + Vulvovaginal Atrophy

44. Transdermal estradiol gel for the treatment of symptomatic postmenopausal women.
45. Bone Levels & Bone Density
46. Dose Levels & Vaginal Atrophy (Patch)

**Chapter Sixteen:**
**Osteoporosis and Restoration of Bone Health**

16.1 Hreshchyshyn MM[1], Hopkins A, Zylstra S, Anbar M. Effects of natural menopause, hysterectomy, and oophorectomy on lumbar spine and femoral neck bone densities.
*Obstet Gynecol.* 1988 Oct;72(4):631-8.

16.2 Imai Y[1], Youn MY, Kondoh S, Nakamura T, Kouzmenko A, Matsumoto T, Takada I, Takaoka K, Kato S. Estrogens maintain bone mass by regulating expression of genes controlling function and life span in mature osteoclasts.
Ann N Y Acad Sci. 2009 Sep;1173 Suppl 1:E31-9. doi: 10.1111/j.1749-6632.2009.04954.x.

16.3 Vanadin Seifert-Klauss[1] and Jerilynn C. Prior[2],* Progesterone and Bone: Actions Promoting Bone Health in Women.
J Osteoporos. 2010; 2010: 845180. Published online 2010 Oct 31. doi: 10.4061/2010/845180. PMCID: PMC2968416 Copyright © 2010 V. Seifert-Klauss and J. C. Prior.

16.4 "The alarming fact is that foods (fruits, vegetables, and grains) now being raised on millions of acres of land that no longer contains enough of certain needed minerals are starving us, no matter how much of them we eat."
—U.S. Senate Document 264. 1936
For an excellent review of food nutrient content see Nutritional Quality of Organically Grown Food by

Steve Diver. Appropriate Technology Transfer for
**(Chapter Sixteen, continued)**
Rural Areas—ATTRA Fayetteville, Arkansas
http://soilandhealth.org/wp-content/uploads/06clip-file/Nutritional%20Quality%20of%20Organically-Grown%20Food.html

**Chapter Seventeen:**
**Weight Issues in Menopause**
17.1 Biochemistry. 5th edition. Section 30.2 Each Organ Has a Unique Metabolic Profile
https://www.ncbi.nlm.nih.gov/books/NBK22436/
17.2 See Appendix B, references 83, 84, and 85
83. Eating behavior and adherence to dietary prescriptions in obese adult subjects treated with 5-hydroxytryptophan.
84. Effects of oral 5-hydroxytryptophan on energy intake and macronutrient selection in non-insulin dependent diabetic patients.
85. 5-hydroxytryptophan: a clinically-effective serotonin precursor.
17.3 See Appendix B, reference 86
86. Tyrosine, phenylalanine, and catecholamine synthesis and function in the brain.

**Chapter Eighteen:**
**In Praise and Honor of the Bladder: Squeeze!**
18.1 By permission, from Nancy Nurge, N.P.

# Appendix A

## 24-Hour Urine Hormone Test Results:
## A Common Example of a Treated Menopausal Woman

Patient:           DOB: 1/12/54  Age: 60  Sex: F  Accession Number

Collection Date: 01/22/14    Date Received:  01/28/14  Physician: DR. DAVED ROSENSWEET
Lab No:               Date Reported:  02/03/14  Test: HORMEST PREG

| TEST | UNITS | ABN | RESULTS | REFERENCE RANGE |
|---|---|---|---|---|
| Estrone (E1) | µg/24hrs | | 5.5 | 1 - 24 µg/24hrs |
| 2-Hydroxyestrone | µg/24hrs | | 6.1 | -- |
| 16-a-Hydroxyestrone | µg/24hrs | | 0.8 | -- |
| 2OH/16OH Estrone ratio | | | 7.6 | -- |

Ratios are likely to be significant only in pre-menopausal or post-menopausal women on HRT who also have levels of E1 that are significantly higher than 5 µg/24hrs. With this in mind, it is generally thought that the ratio of 2OHE1 to 16aOHE1 should be greater than 1 and preferably greater than 2. Post-menopausal women not on HRT generally do not have levels of E1 high enough to produce significant quantities of the hydroxylated metabolites. Also ratios of numbers where the denominator is small may result in misleading interpretations of these ratios.

| TEST | UNITS | ABN | RESULTS | REFERENCE RANGE |
|---|---|---|---|---|
| 4-Hydroxyestrone | µg/24hrs | | 0.4 | -- |

4-OHE1 is a free radical generator and highly estrogenic. As with the other hydroxylated E1 metabolites, levels of 4-OHE1 are likely to be significant only in pre-menopausal or post-menopausal women on HRT who also have levels of E1 greater than approximately 5 µg/24hrs.

| TEST | UNITS | ABN | RESULTS | REFERENCE RANGE |
|---|---|---|---|---|
| Estradiol (E2) | µg/24hrs | | 4.0 | 1 - 26 µg/24hrs |
| Estriol (E3) | µg/24hrs | | 47 | 1 - 63 µg/24hrs |
| Estrogen Ratio | | | 4.9 | - > or =1.0 |
| Total Estrogens | µg/24hrs | | 56 | 3 - 113 µg/24hrs |
| Testosterone | µg/24hrs | | 8.7 | 4 - 18 µg/24hrs |
| Androstanediol | µg/24hrs | | 45 | 15 - 147 µg/24hrs |
| Androstenedione | µg/24hrs | | 1.9 | not established |
| DHEA | µg/24hrs | | 267 | 20 - 1139 µg/24hrs |
| Androstenetriol (5-AT) | µg/24hrs | | 184 | 40 - 540 µg/24hrs |
| Androsterone (AN) | µg/24hrs | | 1002 | 373 - 3414 µg/24hrs |
| 11b-OH-Androsterone (OHAN) | µg/24hrs | | 583 | 201 - 1413 µg/24hrs |
| Etiocholanolone (ET) | µg/24hrs | | 842 | 450 - 2910 µg/24hrs |
| 11b-OH-Etiocholanolone (OHET) | µg/24hrs | | 143 | 33 - 813 µg/24hrs |
| Progesterone | | | NONE DETECTED | - NONE DETECTED |

P is normally not detectable in urine (<<1 µg/24hrs). The level of its major metabolite, ie., pregnanediol, reflects progesterone homeostasis.

| TEST | UNITS | ABN | RESULTS | REFERENCE RANGE |
|---|---|---|---|---|
| Pregnanediol (PD) | µg/24hrs | | 411 | 100 - 3287 µg/24hrs |
| 5-Pregnenetriol (5-PT) | µg/24hrs | | 219 | 44 - 342 µg/24hrs |
| Pregnenolone | | | 0.8 | not established |
| Cortisone (E) | µg/24hrs | | 169 | 49 - 215 µg/24hrs |
| THE | µg/24hrs | | 2143 | 727 - 5788 µg/24hrs |
| THB | µg/24hrs | | 121 | 26 - 262 µg/24hrs |
| THA | µg/24hrs | | 103 | 38 - 298 µg/24hrs |
| Cortisol (F) | µg/24hrs | | 40 | 25 - 115 µg/24hrs |
| THF | µg/24hrs | | 1100 | 458 - 2800 µg/24hrs |
| 5a-THF | µg/24hrs | | 666 | 142 - 2456 µg/24hrs |

NONE DETECTED =< the minimum detectable concentration which is < 1.0 µg/24hrs.
Total Volume = 3900 ml

Patient "feels very good." She was being treated with Bi-Est 30 mg/ml 80:20  (2 drops in the morning and 3 drops in the evening [1.8 mgeeq]).

# Appendix A

## 24-Hour Urine Hormone Test Results
## of an 85-Year-Old Woman
### *Note extremely low hormone levels.*

| TEST | UNITS | ABN | RESULTS | REFERENCE RANGE |
|------|-------|-----|---------|-----------------|
| ESTRONE (E1) | ug/24 hrs | | NONE DETECTED | 1 - 24 ug/24 hrs |
| 2-Hydroxyestrone | ug/24hrs | | NONE DETECTED | --- |
| 16-α-Hydroxyestrone | ug/24hrs | | NONE DETECTED | --- |
| 2OH/16OH Estrone Ratio | | | | --- |

Undefined. Division by zero.

Ratios are likely to be significant only in pre-menopausal or post-menopausal women on HRT who also have levels of E1 that are significantly higher than 5 ug/24 hrs. With this in mind, it is generally thought that the ratio of 2OHE1 to 16αOHE1 should be greater than 1 and preferably greater than 2. Post-menopausal women not on HRT generally do not have levels of E1 high enough to produce significant quantities of the hydroxylated metabolites. Also ratios of numbers where the denominator is small may result in misleading interpretations of these ratios.

| | | | | |
|------|-------|-----|---------|-----------------|
| 4-Hydroxyestrone | ug/24hrs | | NONE DETECTED | --- |

4-OHE1 is a free radical generator and highly estrogenic. As with the other hydroxylated E1 metabolites, levels of 4-OHE1 are likely to be significant only in pre-menopausal or post-menopausal women on HRT who also have levels of E1 greater than approximately 5 ug/24hrs.

| | | | | |
|------|-------|-----|---------|-----------------|
| ESTRADIOL (E2) | ug/24 hrs | LOW | 0.7 | 1 - 26 ug/24 hrs |
| ESTRIOL (E3) | ug/24 hrs | | NONE DETECTED | 1 - 62 ug/24 hrs |
| ESTROGEN RATIO | | | 8 | > or = 1.0 |
| TOTAL ESTROGENS | ug/24 hrs | LOW | 0.7 | 3 - 113 ug/24 hrs |
| TESTOSTERONE | ug/24 hrs | | NONE DETECTED | 4 - 18 ug/24 hrs |
| ANDROSTANEDIOL | ug/24 hrs | LOW | 4 | 15 - 147 ug/24 hrs |
| ANDROSTENEDIONE | ug/24 hrs | | NONE DETECTED | Not Established |
| DHEA | ug/24 hrs | LOW | 19 | 20 - 1139 ug/24 hrs |
| ANDROSTENETRIOL (5-AT) | ug/24 hrs | LOW | 14 | 40 - 540 ug/24 hrs |
| ANDROSTERONE (AN) | ug/24 hrs | LOW | 87 | 373 - 3414 ug/24 hrs |
| 11b-OH Androsterone (OHAN) | ug/24hrs | LOW | 197 | 201 - 1413 ug/24hrs |
| ETIOCHOLANOLONE (ET) | ug/24 hrs | LOW | 171 | 450 - 2910 ug/24 hrs |
| 11b-OH Etiocholanolone (OHET) | ug/24hrs | | 389 | 33 - 813 ug/24hrs |
| PROGESTERONE | | | NONE DETECTED | NONE DETECTED |

P is normally not detectable in urine (<<1 ug/24hrs). The level of its major metabolite, i.e., pregnanediol, reflects progesterone homeostasis.

| | | | | |
|------|-------|-----|---------|-----------------|
| PREGNANEDIOL (PD) | ug/24 hrs | LOW | 16 | 100 - 3287 ug/24 hrs |
| 5-PREGNENETRIOL (5-PT) | ug/24 hrs | LOW | 10 | 44 - 342 ug/24 has |
| PREGNENOLONE | ug/24 hrs | | NONE DETECTED | Not Established |
| CORTISONE (E) | ug/24 hrs | LOW | 43 | 49 - 215 ug/24 hrs |
| THE | ug/24 hrs | | 955 | 727 - 5788 ug/24 hrs |
| TIIB | ug/24 hrs | | 40 | 26 - 262 ug/24 hrs |
| THA | ug/24 hrs | LOW | 27 | 38 - 296 ug/24 hrs |
| CORTISOL (F) | ug/24 hrs | | 39 | 25 - 115 ug/24 hrs |
| THF | ug/24 hrs | LOW | 426 | 458 - 2690 ug/24 hrs |
| 5a-THF | ug/24 hrs | | 325 | 142 - 2456 ug/24 hrs |

None Detected =< the minimum detectable concentration with is <1.0 ug/24hrs.

Total volume = 2150 mL.

# Appendix A

## 24-Hour Urine Hormone Test Results
## of an 89-Year-Old Woman
### *Note extremely low hormone levels.*

Patient:     DOB: 10/28/21  Age: 89  Sex: F  Accession Number: 11-32-006
Collection Date: 01/29/11     Date Received: 02/01/11   Physician: DR. DAVID ROSENSWEET
Lab No: SHP1103522.D          Date Reported: 02/07/11   Test: HORMEST

| TEST | UNITS | ABN | RESULTS | REFERENCE RANGE |
|------|-------|-----|---------|-----------------|
| Estrone (E1) | µg/24hrs | LOW | 0.6 | 1 - 24 µg/24hrs |
| 2-Hydroxyestrone | µg/24hrs | | 1.0 | -- |
| 16-a-Hydroxyestrone | µg/24hrs | | NONE DETECTED | -- |
| 2OH/16OH Estrone ratio | | | Undefined | -- |

Division by zero. Ratios are likely to be significant only in pre-menopausal or post-menopausal women on HRT who also have levels of E1 that are significantly higher than 5 µg/24hrs. With this in mind, it is generally thought that the ratio of 2OH:E1 to 16aOHE1 should be greater than 1 and preferably greater than 2. Post-menopausal women not on HRT generally do not have levels of E1 high enough to produce significant quantities of the hydroxylated metabolites. Also ratios of numbers where the denominator is small may result in misleading interpretations of these ratios.

| | | | | |
|------|-------|-----|---------|-----------------|
| 4-Hydroxyestrone | µg/24hrs | | 0.2 | -- |

4-OHE1 is a free radical generator and highly estrogenic. As with the other hydroxylated E1 metabolites, levels of 4-OHE1 are likely to be significant only in pre-menopausal or post-menopausal women on HRT who also have levels of E1 greater than approximately 5 µg/24hrs.

| | | | | |
|------|-------|-----|---------|-----------------|
| Estradiol (E2) | µg/24hrs | LOW | 0.2 | 1 - 26 µg/24hrs |
| Estriol (E3) | µg/24hrs | | 2.7 | 1 - 63 µg/24hrs |
| Estrogen Ratio | | | 3.1 | - > or =1.0 |
| Total Estrogens | µg/24hrs | | 3.6 | 3 - 113 µg/24hrs |
| Testosterone | µg/24hrs | | NONE DETECTED | 4 - 18 µg/24hrs |
| Androstanediol | µg/24hrs | LOW | 2.9 | 15 - 147 µg/24hrs |
| Androstenedione | µg/24hrs | | NONE DETECTED | not established |
| DHEA | µg/24hrs | LOW | 18 | 20 - 1139 µg/24hrs |
| Androstenetriol (5-AT) | µg/24hrs | LOW | 12 | 40 - 540 µg/24hrs |
| Androsterone (AN) | µg/24hrs | LOW | 147 | 373 - 3414 µg/24hrs |
| 11b-OH-Androsterone (OHAN) | µg/24hrs | LOW | 160 | 201 - 1413 µg/24hrs |
| Etiocholanolone (ET) | µg/24hrs | LOW | 134 | 450 - 3910 µg/24hrs |
| 11b-OH-Etiocholanolone (OHET) | µg/24hrs | | 237 | 33 - 813 µg/24hrs |
| Progesterone | | | NONE DETECTED | - NONE DETECTED |

P is normally not detectable in urine (<<1 µg/24hrs). The level of its major metabolite, i.e., pregnanediol, reflects progesterone homeostasis.

| | | | | |
|------|-------|-----|---------|-----------------|
| Pregnanediol (PD) | µg/24hrs | | 148 | 100 - 3287 µg/24hrs |
| 5-Pregnenetriol (5-PT) | µg/24hrs | LOW | 17 | 44 - 342 µg/24hrs |
| Cortisone (E) | µg/24hrs | | 49 | 49 - 215 µg/24hrs |
| THE | µg/24hrs | | 2287 | 727 - 8788 µg/24hrs |
| THB | µg/24hrs | | 54 | 26 - 262 µg/24hrs |
| THA | µg/24hrs | | 59 | 38 - 298 µg/24hrs |
| Cortisol (F) | µg/24hrs | | 37 | 25 - 115 µg/24hrs |
| THF | µg/24hrs | | 1409 | 458 - 2600 µg/24hrs |
| 5a-THF | µg/24hrs | | 461 | 142 - 2456 µg/24hrs |

COMMENT: INTERPRET WITH CAUTION. NOTE VERY LOW VOLUME.

NONE DETECTED =< the minimum detectable concentration which is < 1.0 µg/24hrs.
Total Volume = 500 ml

# Appendix B

## Select References from the Medical Literature

*Author's note: This section is for those interested in the medical literature and those who would like further citations to back up the material in this book. Happy trails, Dr. R*

### 1. Estrogen and Coronary Artery Disease

Many epidemiological studies show that women who use estrogen therapy after menopause have significantly lower rates of heart disease than postmenopausal women who do not take estrogen. ...the magnitude of the protective effect of estrogen is more pronounced among women with high baseline risk of disease. Estrogen for women at varying risk of coronary disease.
Maturitas. 1998 Sep 20;30(1):19-26.
Grodstein F, Stampfer MJ.

### 2. Cardiovascular and cancer safety of testosterone in women.

Davis SR.
Purpose of Review:
To examine the recent data pertaining to the relationships between testosterone and cardiovascular disease (CVD) and cancer in women.
Recent findings:
Despite the entrenched belief that higher blood levels of testosterone increase the risk of CVD in women, data from recent observational studies mostly show an inverse relationship between testosterone and CVD risk. One pilot study suggests favorable effects of nonoral testosterone treatment of women with established congestive cardiac failure which merits further evaluation. The relationship between endogenous testosterone production and breast cancer risk remains contentious, with recent studies indicating either no relationship, or a possible increase in risk when estrone and estradiol are not taken into account. No randomized controlled trial of testosterone therapy has been sufficiently large or of sufficient duration to establish whether such treatment may influence breast cancer occurrence. There does not appear to be an association between testosterone and endometrial cancer, or other malignancies on review of published studies.
Summary:

Testosterone is inversely associated with increased CVD risk in women, whereas low sex hormone binding globulin increases CVD risk. The relationship between testosterone and breast cancer remains unclear, although a clear signal of risk has not emerged from studies of women treated with testosterone therapy over the past decade.
Curr Opin Endocrinol Diabetes Obes. 2011 Jun;18(3):198-203. doi: 10.1097/ MED.0b013e328344f449.

### 3. Estrogen and Memory

The existence of estrogen receptors in the hippocampus, a part of the brain essential to learning and memory, has been known for some time46. Several mechanisms may account for the effects of estrogen on the brain. Firstly, estrogen increases levels of choline O-acetyl- transferase, the enzyme needed to synthesize acetylcholine, a neurotransmitter thought to be critical for memory47. Studies on healthy middle-aged and elderly postmenopausal women have supported the theory that estrogen may help to maintain aspects of cognitive function 48,49. Data also suggest that estrogen replacement therapy may enhance short- and long-term memory 50,51. Additional effects of estrogen on neural function include: protecting neurons from oxidative stress and glutamate toxicity [89,90], increasing glucose transport and cerebral blood flow [91], and stimulating the branching of neurites [91].
Michelle P. Warren, M.D. and Jennifer E. Dominguez, B.A. www.endotext. com., Updated 5 January 2004

### 4. Estrogen and Alzheimer's Disease

For every five years after the age of 65, the prevalence of Alzheimer's disease doubles in the population. Nearly 50% of women over the age of 75 may suffer from the condition52. As the population ages over the next 20 years, these numbers are expected to increase. According to epidemiologic evidence, there is reason to believe that estrogen deficiency may contribute to Alzheimer's disease. Low body weight is associated with low levels of circulating estrogens in postmenopausal women. Women who suffer from Alzheimer's disease tend to have lower body weights than women without the disorder. Incidences of Alzheimer's disease are low or its expression is delayed in postmenopausal women with high levels of endogenous estrogenic steroids or those receiving long-term HRT.
Michelle P. Warren, M.D. and Jennifer E. Dominguez, B.A. www.endotext. com., Updated 5 January 2004

### 5. HRT and Weight Gain

Because many women gain weight as they age, a common fear is that HRT will exacerbate this problem. However, this is unconfirmed by prospective studies. The PEPI trial showed that women on HRT gained less weight than women not taking hormones. Attention to diet (with reduced fat intake) and regular aerobic exercise for weight maintenance should be recommended to all post-menopausal women.

Michelle P. Warren, M.D. and Jennifer E. Dominguez, B.A. www.endotext. com., Updated 5 January 2004

### 6. Estrogen Dose Levels and Bone Density

...we investigated the safety and effectiveness in preventing bone loss of, very-low-dose estradiol [0.014 mg/d] transdermal unopposed for postmenopausal women  (n = 208)

Conclusion: Postmenopausal treatment with low-dose, unopposed estradiol increased bone mineral density and decreased markers of bone turnover without causing endometrial hyperplasia.

Obstet Gynecol. 2004 Sep;104(3):443-51.

Effects of ultralow-dose transdermal estradiol on bone mineral density: a randomized clinical trial.     Ettinger B, Ensrud KE, et al.

### 7. Estrogen Neuroprotection and the Critical Period Hypothesis [Review article]

In summary, 17β-estradiol is an endogenous steroid hormone produced primarily by the ovaries, which has the ability to attenuate damage from cerebral ischemia and delay onset of cognitive decline in both animals and humans. Furthermore, high levels of serum E2 can partially explain women's relative protection from heart attacks, strokes, and neurodegenerative diseases until late in life..Despite overwhelming evidence of the neuroprotective and cardioprotective functions of estradiol and the dire consequences of long-term E2 deprivation...merging evidence from basic science and clinical studies, which suggests that there is a "critical period" for estradiol's beneficial effect in the brain [peri-menopause]

Erin Scott, Quan-guang Zhang et al. Front Neuroendocrinol.2012 January:33(1): 85-104.

### 8. Breast Cancer Risk: Mainstream View

One in 8 women will be diagnosed with breast cancer and risk increases with age.

Estrogen, a trophic growth hormone, may promote the growth of preexisting breast cancer.

It is still unknown whether it may also induce the growth of new cancers.

Use of Estrogen alone for at least five years, may be associated with a slightly increased risk of breast cancer according to the Nurses' Health Study.

Reprinted from www.Endotext.com

Michelle Warren, M.D. and Aimee Shu M.D.•Updated September 2010

### 9. Estrogen: Breast Cancer, Trophic or Initiator?

Estrogen, a trophic growth hormone, may promote the growth of preexisting breast cancer.

It is still unknown whether it may also induce the growth of new cancers.

However, in the recent report from the Women's Health Initiative study, women on estrogen only showed no increased incidences of breast cancer compared to women on placebo

Many studies have not shown an increased risk of breast cancer with estrogen use.

A large meta-analysis of 51 epidemiologic studies (involving more than 160,000 women from 21 countries) showed that HRT[CEE + Progestin(?)] increases the risk of breast cancer and that risk increases with longer use. That is, for every 1,000 women who began using HRT at age 50 and continued using it for 5, 10, or 15 years, an additional 2, 6, or 12 cases of breast cancer occurred. Reprinted from Endotext.org. Michelle Warren, M.D. and Aimee Shu M.D. Updated September 2010

### 10. Women's Health Initiative (WHI) and the issues related to it

Recent evidence suggests, however, that estrogen plus progestin may have an impact on breast cancer. In July 2002, the estrogen plus progestin arm of the Women's Health Initiative study was stopped due to a small increase in the incidence of breast cancer among women taking this combination. This risk amounted to approximately 8 more women per 10,000 being diagnosed with breast cancer compared to those on placebo. (66) It is important to note, however, that the average age of women in this study was 63.2 years, and does not reflect women on HRT in normal clinical practice. In addition, 50% of the women in WHI were either current or former smokers, they had an average BMI of 28 (well-above normal), and 1/3 suffered from hypertension.

### 11. Hormone Treatment and Breast Cancer Risk

Re the two arms of the WHI study

The average risk of invasive breast cancer with estrogen use was 0.79...[while] The average breast cancer risk with estrogen-progestin use was 1.24

Collins JA, et al. Hum Reprod Update. 2005 Nov-Dec;11(6):541-3.Review article Breast cancer risk with postmenopausal hormonal treatment.

**12. The incidence of breast cancer and changes in the use of hormone replacement therapy: A review of the evidence.**

A considerable amount of scientific evidence supports the hypothesis that the decline in the incidence of breast cancer is in large part attributable to the sudden drop in HRT use following publication of the WHI and Million Women studies.

Maturitas. 2009 Aug 24.

Verkooijen HM, Bouchardy C, Vinh-Hung V, Rapiti E, Hartman M.

**13a. Relative Risk of Heart Disease vs Breast Cancer in Women**

Women's age-adjusted mortality rates from heart disease are four to six times higher than their mortality rates from breast cancer. Yet, because public campaigns have emphasized breast cancer risks in the effort to promote screening mammography, many women are more afraid of breast cancer than of coronary artery disease....

When women present with myocardial infarction, they are more likely than men to be misdiagnosed, and they are also more likely to die of their first infarction

Women present at a later age

Coronary Artery Disease Prevention: What's Different for Women? J Bedinghaus M.D. L LeShan M.D.et, al. Medical College of Wisconsin, Milwaukee, Wisconsin

Am Fam Physician. 2001 Apr 1;63(7):1393-1401.

**13b. Relationship between Menopausal Symptoms and Risk of Postmenopausal Breast Cancer**

Results: Women who ever experienced menopausal symptoms had lower risks of invasive ductal carcinoma [(IDC) OR = 0.5; 95% CI: 0.3–0.7], invasive lobular carcinoma (ILC, OR = 0.5; 95% CI: 0.3–0.8), and invasive ductal-lobular carcinoma (IDLC, OR = 0.7; 95% CI: 0.4–1.2), and these reductions in risk were independent of recency and timing of hormone therapy use, age at menopause, and body mass index. Increasing intensity of hot flushes among women who ever experienced hot flushes was also associated with decreasing risks of all three breast cancer subtypes (P values for trend all ≤0.017).

Conclusion:

This is the first study to report that women who ever experienced menopausal symptoms have a substantially reduced risk of breast cancer, and that severity of hot flushes is also inversely associated with risk.

Yi Huang1, Kathleen E. Malone1 et al

Cancer Epidemiol Biomarkers Prev 2011;20:379-388.
http://cebp.aacrjournals.org/content/20/2/379.full.pdf+html

### 14. Urinary estrogens and estrogen metabolites and subsequent risk of breast cancer among premenopausal women.

Higher urinary estrone and estradiol levels were strongly significantly associated with lower risk....

Generally inverse, although nonsignificant, patterns also were observed with 2- and 4-hydroxylation pathway estrogen metabolites. Inverse associations generally were not observed with 16-pathway estrogen metabolites and a significant positive association was observed with 17-epiestriol The inverse associations with parent estrogen metabolites and the parent estrogen metabolite/non-parent estrogen metabolite ratio suggest that women with higher urinary excretion of parent estrogens are at lower risk.

Eliassen AH, Spiegelman D, Xu X,
Cancer Res; 72(3); 696–706. ©2011

### 15. Mammographic density and estrogen receptor status of breast cancer.

Results: Mammographic density was strongly associated with both ER-positive and ER-negative breast cancers. Cancer Epidemiology, Biomarkers & Prevention December 2004 13; 2090

Conclusion: Surprisingly, women with high mammographic density have an increased risk of both ER-positive and ER-negative breast cancers. The association between mammographic density and breast cancer may be due to factors besides estrogen exposure.

### 16. Circulating Steroid Hormone Levels and Risk of Breast Cancer for Postmenopausal Women.

Cancer Epidemiol Biomarkers Prev; 19(2); 492–502.

Our prospective study confirms earlier findings and suggests that the associations of endogenous hormones with postmenopausal breast cancer risk are independent of tumor grade, and hormone receptor status and might increase in strength with age.

### 17. Circulating sex steroids and breast cancer risk in premenopausal women.

Recently, the associations between circulating hormones in premenopausal women and subsequent risk of breast cancer have been evaluated. To date, both positive and null associations have been observed for estrogens and inverse and null associations for progesterone with breast cancer risk. For estrogens, the relationships may vary by menstrual cycle phase (e.g., follicular versus

luteal phase), although this requires confirmation. Few studies have evaluated estrogen metabolites in relation to breast cancer risk; hence, no conclusions can yet be drawn. Findings for the largely adrenal-derived dehydroepiandrosterone (DHEA) and DHEA sulfate also are inconsistent and may vary by age. However, relatively consistent positive associations have been observed between testosterone (or free testosterone) levels and breast cancer risk; these associations are of similar magnitude to those confirmed among postmenopausal women. In this review, we summarize current evidence and identify gaps and inconsistencies that need to be addressed in future studies of sex steroids and premenopausal breast cancer risk. Horm Cancer. 2010 Feb;1(1):2-10. doi: 10.1007/s12672-009-0003-0. Epub 2010 Feb 9.
Source. Susan E. Hankinson & A. Heather Eliassen
Channing Laboratory, Department of Medicine, Harvard Medical School and Brigham and Women's Hospital,

### 18. Modern Menstruation
One hundred years ago, the average woman started her menses at age 16. She got pregnant earlier and more frequently. She often spent more time lactating. In total, women back then experienced the menstrual cycle about 100 to 200 times in their lifetime. Today, the average modern women starts puberty at age 12, seldom lactates, has less children, and menstruates about 350 to 400 times during a lifetime. Incessant menstruation has been associated with the increased occurrence of a myriad of pathological conditions including infertility, cancer, fibroids, anemia, migraines, mood shifts, abdominal pain, fluid retention, and endometriosis. What a difference a century makes!
Michael Lam M.D.
http://www.drlam.com/articles/estrogen_dominance.asp

### 19. Urinary estrogens and estrogen metabolites and subsequent risk of breast cancer among premenopausal women.
Abstract: Endogenous estrogens and estrogen metabolism are hypothesized to be associated with premenopausal breast cancer risk but evidence is limited. We examined 15 urinary estrogens/ estrogen metabolites (EM) and breast cancer risk among premenopausal women in a case-control study nested within the Nurses' Health Study II (NHSII). In 1996–1999, urine was collected from 18,521 women during the mid-luteal menstrual phase. Breast cancer cases (N=247) diagnosed between collection and June 2005 were matched to 2 controls each (N=485). Urinary EM were measured by liquid chromatography-tandem mass spectrometry and adjusted for creatinine level. Relative risks (RRs) and 95% confidence intervals (CIs) were estimated by multivariate conditional logistic regression. Higher urinary estrone and estradiol levels

were strongly significantly associated with lower risk (top vs. bottom quartile RR estrone=0.52, 95% CI=(0.30– 0.88); estradiol=0.51, 95% CI=(0.30–0.86)). Generally inverse, though non-significant, patterns also were observed with 2- and 4-hydroxylation pathway EM. Inverse associations generally were not observed with 16-pathway EM and a significant positive association was observed with 17- epiestriol (top vs. bottom quartile RR=1.74, 95% CI=(1.08–2.81), p-trend=0.01). In addition, there was a significant increased risk with higher 16-pathway/parent EM ratio (comparable RR=1.61, 95% CI=(0.99–2.62), p-trend=0.04). Other pathway ratios were not significantly associated with risk except parent EM/non-parent EM (comparable RR=0.58, 95% CI=(0.35–0.96), p-trend=0.03). These data suggest that most mid-luteal urinary EM concentrations are not positively associated with breast cancer risk among premenopausal women. The inverse associations with parent EM and the parent EM/non-parent EM ratio suggest that women with higher urinary excretion of parent estrogens are at lower risk.

A. Heather Eliassen1,3, Donna Spiegelman3,4, Xia Xu, et. al. Cancer Res. 2012 February 1; 72(3): 696–706. doi:10.1158/0008-5472.CAN-11-2507.

### 20. The Mortality Toll of Estrogen Avoidance: An Analysis of Excess Deaths Among Hysterectomized Women Aged 50 to 59 Years [courtesy of Eugene Shippen M.D.]

Objectives. We examined the effect of estrogen avoidance on mortality rates among hysterectomized women aged 50 to 59 years.

Methods. We derived a formula to relate the excess mortality among hysterectomized women aged 50 to 59 years assigned to placebo in the Women's Health Initiative randomized controlled trial to the entire population of comparable women in the United States, incorporating the decline in estrogen use observed between 2002 and 2011.

Results. Over a 10-year span, starting in 2002, a minimum of 18 601 and as many as 91 610 postmenopausal women died prematurely because of the avoidance of estrogen therapy (ET).

Conclusions. ET in younger postmenopausal women is associated with a decisive reduction in all-cause mortality, but estrogen use in this population is low and continuing to fall. Our data indicate an associated annual mortality toll in the thousands of women aged 50 to 59 years. Informed discussion between these women and their health care providers about the effects of ET is a matter of considerable urgency.

Philip M. Sarrel, MD, et al. Am J Public Health. 2013.301295). http://ajph.aphapublications.org/doi/abs/10.2105/AJPH.2013.301295.

### 21. Holtorf's Review: Are Bio-identical Hormones Safer or More Efficacious?

This literature review presents the substantial evidence for the safety and efficacy of bio-identical hormone therapy, including estradiol, estriol, and progesterone, which shows that it presents lower risks for breast cancer and cardiovascular disease than synthetic or animal-derived hormones. Studies show that progestins have a number of negative effects on the cardiovascular system and an association with breast cancer risk that can be avoided by using bioidentical progesterone.

The Bioidentical Hormone Debate: Are Bioidentical Hormones (Estradiol, Estriol, and Progesterone) Safer or More Efficacious than Commonly Used Synthetic Versions in Hormone Replacement Therapy?

Holtorf K   Postgrad Med 2009;121(1):1-13..

### 22. Transdermal Hormone Rx & Risk

In conclusion, while all types of hormone replacement therapies are safe and effective and confer significant benefits in the long-term when initiated in young postmenopausal women, in specific clinical settings the choice of the transdermal route of administration of estrogens and the use of natural progesterone might offer significant benefits and added safety.

Could transdermal estradiol + progesterone be a safer postmenopausal HRT? A review.

Maturitas. 2008 Jul-Aug;60(3-4):185-201. Epub 2008 Sep 5

L'hermite M, Simoncini T, Fuller S, Genazzani AR.Department of Gynecology and Obstetrics, Université Libre de Bruxelles, Bruxelles, Belgium.

### 23. Unequal risks for breast cancer associated with different hormone replacement therapies: results from the E3N cohort study.

This large multicenter study in France followed 80,377 postmenopausal women for up to 12 years, and looked in particular at whether the type of progestogen used in combination with estrogen made a difference to the risk of developing breast cancer in those women who used hormone replacement therapy (HRT). The estrogen in HRT is primarily transdermal estradiol in France. Compared with those women who did not use HRT at all, women using estrogen alone had a 1.29-fold increased risk of developing breast cancer; women using estrogen plus natural progesterone had the same risk as women using no HRT.

Unequal risks for breast cancer associated with different hormone replacement therapies: results from the E3N cohort study.

Breast Cancer Res Treat 2008;107(1):103-11.

Fournier A, Berrino F, Clavel-Chapelon F.

### 24. Breast Cancer Risk and the 2 Estrogen Receptors

...It has turned out that estrogen action is not mediated by one receptor, ERalpha, but by two balancing factors, ERalpha and ERbeta, which are often antagonistic to one another. Excitingly, ERbeta has been shown to be widespread in the body and to be involved in a multitude of physiological and pathophysiological events. This has led to a strong interest of the pharmaceutical industry to target ERbeta by drugs against various diseases. In this review, focus is on the role of ERbeta in malignant diseases where the anti proliferative activity of ERbeta gives hope of new therapeutic approaches.

The role of estrogen receptor beta (ERbeta) in malignant diseases--a new potential target for antiproliferative drugs in prevention and treatment of cancer. Biochem Biophys Res Commun. 2010 May 21;396(1):63-6.

Warner M, Gustafsson JA. Department of BioSciences and Nutrition, Karolinska Institutet, Stockholm, Sweden.

### 25. Estriol preferentially binds to ERβ

...we studied the binding affinities of... more than 50 steroidal analogs of estradiol-17β (E2) and estrone (E1) for human ERα and ERβ... several of the D-ring metabolites, such as 16α-hydroxyestradiol (estriol),... , had distinct preferential binding affinity for human ERβ over ERα (difference up to 18-fold). Notably, although E2 has nearly the highest and equal binding affinity for ERα and ERβ, E1 and 2-hydroxyestrone... have preferential binding affinity for ERα over ERβ, whereas 16α-hydroxyestradiol (estriol)... have preferential binding affinity for ERβ over ERα

Quantitative Structure-Activity Relationship of Various Endogenous Estrogen Metabolites for Human Estrogen Receptor α and β Subtypes: Insights into the Structural Determinants Favoring a Differential Subtype Binding.
Endocrinology Zhu et al. September 2006 147 (9): 4132

### 26. Estriol generates tolerogenic dendritic cells in vivo that protect against autoimmunity.

Chronic inflammation contributes to numerous diseases, and regulation of inflammation is crucial for disease control and resolution. Sex hormones have potent immunoregulatory abilities. Specifically, estrogen influences immune cells and inflammation, which contributes to the sexual dimorphism of autoimmunity and protection against disease seen during pregnancy in multiple sclerosis (MS) and its animal model, experimental autoimmune encephalomyelitis (EAE). Although long thought to act primarily on T cells, recent evidence demonstrated that myeloid cells, such as dendritic cells (DCs), are essential in mediating estrogen's protective effects. Estriol (E3), a pregnancy-specific estrogen, has therapeutic efficacy in MS and EAE, and we evaluated whether E3 could act exclusively through DCs to protect against the inflammatory autoimmune disease EAE. Levels of activation markers (CD80 and CD86) and inhibitory co-stimulatory markers (PD-L1, PD-L2, B7–H3, and B7–H4) were increased in E3 DCs. E3 DCs had decreased proinflammatory IL-12, IL-23, and IL-6 mRNA expression, increased immunoregulatory IL-10 and TGF-β mRNA expression, and a decreased ratio of IL-12/IL-10 protein production. Importantly, transfer of E3 DCs to mice prior to active induction of EAE protected them from developing EAE through immune deviation to a Th2 response. This protection was apparent, even in the face of in vitro and in vivo inflammatory challenge. In summary, our results showed that E3 generates tolerogenic DCs, which protect against the inflammatory autoimmune disease EAE. Targeted generation of tolerogenic DCs with immunomodulatory therapeutics, such as E3, has potential applications in the treatment of numerous autoimmune and chronic inflammatory diseases.

J Immunol. 2011 March 15; 186(6): 3346–3355. Tracey L. Papenfuss, Nicole D. Powell

### 27. Hormone replacement therapy and breast density changes.

Objectives: To compare the incidence of increased breast density and tenderness in postmenopausal women associated with transdermal (Estalis/Combipatch®, Novartis, Basel, Switzerland) and oral (Kliogest®, Schering AG, Berlin, Germany) hormone replacement therapy (HRT).

Methods   A total of 202 postmenopausal women were randomized to transdermal or oral HRT. Mammograms obtained at study entry and after 1 year of treatment were assessed for percent breast density by means of the digital segmentation and thresholding technique. Breast tenderness was assessed at each study visit.

Results   The mean breast density by ANCOVA after adjusting for screening value at study end was significantly lower for women using Estalis® (38.4%, standard error 0.9%) compared with Kliogest® (46.9%, standard error 1.5%) (p<0.0001). Significantly fewer women using transdermal HRT had an increase in mammographic breast density or breast tenderness compared to oral HRT. Of the women using transdermal HRT, 39.1% had no change in breast density compared to 15.7% for women using oral HRT. Only 4% of women using transdermal HRT had a marked increase in density (>25%) compared to 15.7% of women using oral HRT. Overall, 36.0% of patients in the transdermal group reported breast tenderness at some point during the 1-year study, compared with 57.6% in the oral HRT group (p=0.0002).

Conclusion   Transdermal HRT use is associated with a significantly lower incidence of increased mammographic breast density and breast tenderness compared with oral HRT.

Climacteric. J Harvey, C Scheurer, et al. 2005 Jun;8(2):185-92.  2005, Vol. 8, No. 2 , Pages 185-192

### 28. Are all estrogens created equal?

A review of oral vs. transdermal therapy.

Abstract

Background:

To compare oral and transdermal delivery systems in domains of lipid effects; cardiovascular, inflammatory, and thrombotic effects; effect on insulin-like growth factor, insulin resistance, and metabolic syndrome; sexual effects; metabolic effects including weight; and effects on target organs bone, breast, and uterus. Methods:

Review of the literature 1990-2010. Studies selected on basis of applicability, quality of data, and relationship to topic. Results: Data applicable to the comparisons of oral versus transdermal delivery systems for postmenopausal estrogen therapy were utilized to perform a review and formulate conclusions.

Conclusions:

Significant differences appear to exist between oral and transdermal estrogens in terms of hormonal bioavailability and metabolism, with implications for clinical efficacy, potential side effects, and risk profile of different hormone therapy options, but neither results nor study designs are uniform. Bypassing hepatic metabolism appears to result in more stable serum estradiol levels without supraphysiologic concentrations in the liver. By avoiding first-pass metabolism, transdermal hormone therapy may have less pronounced effects on hepatic protein synthesis, such as inflammatory markers, markers of coagulation and fibrinolysis, and steroid binding proteins, while oral hormone therapy has more pronounced hyper-coagulant effects and increases synthesis of C-reactive protein and fibrinolytic markers. Both oral and transdermal delivery systems have beneficial effects on high-density lipoprotein cholesterol to low-density lipoprotein cholesterol ratios (oral>transdermal), while the transdermal system has more favorable effects on triglycerides. Incidence of metabolic syndrome and weight gain appears to be slightly lower with a transdermal delivery system. Oral estrogen's significant increase in hepatic sex hormone binding globulin production lowers testosterone availability compared with transdermal delivery, with clinically relevant effects on sexual vigor.

Goodman MP. J Womens Health (Larchmt). 2012 Feb;21(2):161-9. doi: 10.1089/jwh.2011.2839. Epub 2011 Oct 19.

### 29. Oral Estrogen: Metabolite, Coagulation, and Other Issues

•Oral estradiol leads to higher 2-hydroxyestrone and 16α-hydroxyestrone metabolites

•Also, can occur in previous premarin users!!!

•Oral estradiol raises estrone when metabolized by CytP450 enzymes and hence changes estrone, estradiol and estriol ratio (estrogen quotient)

•Oral estriol increased the relative risk of endometrial neoplasia, whereas vaginal application did not

•Oral HRT containing estradiol is associated with a marked and rapid increase in CRP
[relates to thrombosis risk]
•Oral estradiol increases the mean value of prothrombin activation peptide and decreases mean antithrombin activity
•Oral estradiol associated with a significant decrease in mean tissue-type plasminogen concentration and plasminogen activator inhibitor activity and a significant rise in global fibrinolytic capacity
Christina Hinchcliffe N.D.


### 30. Coagulation Issues Matter
Women's age-adjusted mortality rates from heart disease are four to six times higher than their mortality rates from breast cancer.
Coronary Artery Disease Prevention: What's Different for Women? J Bedinghaus M.D. L LeShan M.D.et, al. Medical College of Wisconsin, Milwaukee, Wisconsin
Am Fam Physician. 2001 Apr 1;63(7):1393-1401.


### 31. Oral Estrogen and the Gall Bladder
The risk of cholecystectomy was increased among women exposed to oral estrogen menopausal hormone therapy, especially oral regimens without a progestagen.
Complicated gallstone disease should be added to the list of potential adverse events to be considered when balancing the benefits and risks associated with menopausal hormone therapy.
Menopausal hormone therapy and risk of cholecystectomy: a prospective study based on the French E3N. Antoine Racine, MD MSc, Anne Bijon, MSc, Agnès Fournier, PhD, CMAJ. 2013 April 16; 185(7): 555–561.
http://www.ncbi.nlm.nih.gov/pmc/articles/PMC3626807/


### 32. Oral Estradiol: Increased Hormone & Metabolite Issues
Conclusion: The previously recommended oral dose of estradiol (1-2mg/day) results in urinary excretion of estrone at values 5-10 times the upper limit of the reference range for premenopausal women. Retrospective studies associating oral estradiol with increased risk of breast cancer may reflect overdose conditions. Based on current knowledge, a prudent dose ceiling for oral estradiol replacement therapy of 0.25mg/day is proposed.
Wright, JV, Friel, P, Hinchcliffe, C: Hormone Replacement with Estradiol: Conventional Oral Doses result in Excessive Exposure to Estrone. Alternative Medicine Review: Vol 10, Num 1 2005

### 33. Transdermal vs Oral Estrogen: Another Resource

Since there is no first-pass liver deactivation of transdermal estradiol, effective doses are small. First-pass metabolism of oral estradiol is associated with adverse events traditionally attributed to menopausal hormone therapy. First pass significantly impairs bioavailability of oral estradiol. Large doses required to overcome first pass induce supraphysiologic release of hepatic proteins, including C-reactive protein (CRP), insulin-like growth factor 1, clotting factors, and hormone-binding globulins (ie, sex hormone–binding globulin [SHBG], thyroxine-binding globulin [TBG], and cortisol-binding globulin [CBG]).1-3 First pass impacts adversely on lipids, cardiovascular functions, inflammatory and thrombotic mechanisms, insulin resistance, and weight control, and it may aggravate metabolic syndrome.

John E. Buster, MD Professor of Obstetrics and Gynecology,

### 34. Premarin

"Premarin is one of the all-time best-selling prescription drugs, and it had global sales of more than $2 billion in 2001. But the health concerns raised by the WHI study have had an impact on sales, which dropped to $880 million in 2004". Chemical and Engineering News

http://pubs.acs.org/cen/coverstory/83/8325/8325premarin.html

### 35. Premarin

CDER concludes that the reference listed drug Premarin is not adequately characterized at this time. In particular, the estrogenic potency of the product is not clearly defined relative to the estrogenic potency of its constituents. In addition, the contribution of the two most abundant estrogens, sodium equilin sulfate and sodium estrone sulfate, to the overall estrogenic potency is not well understood. Furthermore, the quantitative composition of Premarin with respect to potentially pharmacologically active components has not been defined. Without this information, it is not possible to define the active ingredients of Premarin.

Source: U.S. FDA FDA Backgrounder on Conjugated Estrogens 2005

http://www.fda.gov/Drugs/DrugSafety/InformationbyDrugClass/ucm168838.htm

### 36. Carbopol ("Carbomer," etc.) Carbopol and its Pharmaceutical Significance: A Review

"Carbopol polymers are polymers of acrylic acid cross-linked with polyalkenyl ethers or divinyl glycol...carboxyvinyl polymer, carboxy polymethylene, carboxy polymethylene..."

http://www.oalib.com/paper/2260424#.WcaZv0yZNE4

### 37. Propylene Glycol Toxicity

Conclusion: Propylene glycol toxicity is a potentially life-threatening iatrogenic complication that is common and preventable. It should be considered whenever a patient has an unexplained anion gap, unexplained metabolic acidosis, hyperosmolality, and/or clinical deterioration. Close monitoring of all patients receiving IV lorazepam or diazepam for early evidence of propylene glycol toxicity is warranted......

Despite the reputation of propylene glycol for safety, propylene glycol toxicity has been reported. Adverse effects from propylene glycol have occurred when used to deliver topical sulfadiazine silver cream,345 IV nitroglycerine,6 etomidate,7 enoximone,8 multivitamins,910

Wilson M.D. et. al. Chest. September 2005 vol128 #3 1674-1681

### 38. The temporal reliability of serum estrogens, progesterone, gonadotropins, SHBG and urinary estrogen and progesterone metabolites in premenopausal

*women.*This study confirms previous findings that SHBG may be reliably measured in premenopausal women using a single occasion. It also indicates that E1S may be reliably measured using one sample only. More importantly, our results suggest that none of the (Estradiol, Progesterone, SHBG, FSH, LH other analytes examined meet minimal reliability requirements that would permit confidence in single measures. These results are in agreement with the wide range if ICCs reported in previous studies [4-6]. Our conclusions are limited to the collection of samples at midluteal phase, however, and may not generalize to other phases of the menstrual cycle.

Andrew E Williams, Gertraud Maskarinec, Adrian A Franke and Frank Z Stanczyk. BMC Women's Health 2002, 2:13
23 December 2002

### 39. 2-OH/16a-OH: Risk Reduction

Risk for breast cancer includes decreased 2OH/16aOH, increased testosterone, deficiency of estriol, and insufficient progesterone. Brassica's, DIM, can be beneficial to reduce risks as well as a lower prolactin being risk reducing.

Reducing the Hormone Related Cancer Risk
(Or cabbages, sex hormones and their metabolites).
By Jonathan Wright MD: Nutrition and Healing
https://www.antiaging-systems.com/articles/129-cancer-risk-reduction

### 40. Estrogen Metabolite Ratio Reaffirmed

...In conclusion, we have shown that
the preponderance of evidence from the study of estrogen metabolites in tissues

and urine supports the EMR [estrogen metabolite ratio] hypothesis,
and that the EMR can be modulated in a predictable manner through dietary
changes and use of certain nutraceuticals.
Response to Dr. Jacob Schor's Article 'Estrogen Metabolite Ratios: Time for
Us to Let Go' Thomas Klug PhD Townsend Letter. April 2013. p100 – 106.

### 41. Relationship of serum estrogens and estrogen metabolites to postmeno-pausal breast cancer risk: a nested case-control study.

Conclusions: Women with more extensive hydroxylation along the 2-pathway
may have a reduced risk of postmenopausal breast cancer. Further studies are
needed to clarify the risks for specific EM and complex patterns of estrogen
metabolism. This will require aggregation of EM results from several studies.
Roni T Falk (falkr@mail.nih.gov) Louise A Brinton
Breast Cancer Research 2013, 15:R34

### 42. Cancer Growth vs Initiation

The development of cancer from the first malignant tumour cell to clinical
diagnosis takes many years. Hormones can influence tumour growth, but it is
questionable whether hormones induce malignant tumours de novo. It is much
more likely that hormones 'merely' promote the growth of already existing
tumour cells.
Hormone replacement therapy: pathobiological aspects
of hormone-sensitive cancers in women relevant to
epidemiological studies on HRT: a mini-review
Human Reproduction Vol.20, No.8 pp. 2052–2060, 2005
M.Dietel1,4, M.A.Lewis2 and S.Shapiro3

### 43. Transdermal estradiol gel 0.1% for the treatment of vasomotor symptoms in postmenopausal women.

Low Dose TD Carbopol Gel Improves  HF + Vulvovaginal Atrophy
Objective: The objective of this study was to evaluate the efficacy and safety
of three doses of estradiol gel 0.1% (Divigel, a novel formulation consisting of
1 mg estradiol per 1 g transdermal gel) to reduce the frequency and severity of
vasomotor symptoms and signs of vulvar and vaginal atrophy associated with
menopause.
Conclusions: Low-dose transdermal estradiol gel 0.1% is an effective treatment for relief of vasomotor symptoms, as well as signs of vulvar and vaginal
atrophy, associated with menopause. Estradiol gel 0.1% offers multiple dosing
options to individualize patient therapy, including the
lowest available effective dose (0.25 mg estradiol, delivering 0.003 mg/d estra-

diol) to treat the vasomotor symptoms of menopause.
Hedrick, et al. 2009-01, Menopause., 16(1):132-40

### 44. Transdermal estradiol gel for the treatment of symptomatic postmeno-pausal women.

Abstract
Objective: The aim of this study was to determine the efficacy, safety, and lowest practical dose of a transdermal estradiol gel in the treatment of symptomatic postmenopausal women.
Methods: Healthy postmenopausal women with seven or more moderate to severe hot flushes per day or 50 to 60 or more per week were randomized to transdermal gel containing 1.5 mg (n = 73) or 0.75 mg (n = 75) estradiol (EstroGel 0.06%) or placebo (n = 73) in a phase 3 study, or to 0.375 mg (n = 119) or 0.27 mg (n = 118) estradiol (0.03% gel) or placebo (n = 114) in a phase 4 study.
Results: The frequency of moderate to severe hot flushes and severity of all hot flushes significantly decreased versus placebo at weeks 4 and 12 with 1.5, 0.75, and 0.375 mg estradiol. Overall participant responder rates were generally lower in the phase 4 study than those in the phase 3 study with the approved 0.75-mg estradiol dose. Vaginal maturation index (VMI) shifts from baseline to week 12 were significant (P < 0.001) with 0.75 and 1.5 mg estradiol versus placebo; VMI improved (P < 0.001), superficial cells increased (P = 0.005), and parabasal cells decreased (P = 0.002) with 0.375 mg estradiol vs placebo but not with 0.27 mg estradiol. CONCLUSION: A transdermal gel with 0.75 mg estradiol was the lowest practical dose that effectively reduced the frequency and severity of moderate to severe hot flushes, improved VMI [Vaginal Maturation Index], and was well tolerated.
Archer DF, et al.   Menopause. 2012 Jun;19(6):622-9.

### 45. Dose Levels & Bone Density
…we investigated the safety and effectiveness in preventing bone loss of, very-low-dose estradiol [0.014 mg/d][delivered] transdermal unopposed for post-menopausal women  (n = 208)
Conclusion: Postmenopausal treatment with low-dose, unopposed estradiol increased bone mineral density and decreased markers of bone turnover without causing endometrial hyperplasia.
Obstet Gynecol. 2004 Sep;104(3):443-51.
Effects of ultralow-dose transdermal estradiol on bone mineral density: a randomized clinical trial.
Ettinger B, Ensrud KE, et al.

### 46. Dose Levels & Vaginal Atrophy: (patch)

Conclusion: During 2 years of treatment with ultralow- dose [ultra-low dose: 14mcg patch] unopposed estradiol, treatment and placebo groups had similar rates of endometrial hyperplasia, endometrial proliferation, and vaginal bleeding. This therapy apparently causes little or no endometrial stimulation....Vaginal epithelial cells showed greater maturation in the estradiol group than in the placebo group (P < .001) but less than typically observed with standard doses of estrogen.

Uterine and Vaginal Effects of Unopposed Ultralow- Dose Transdermal Estradiol. OBSTETRICS & GYNECOLOGY. VOL. 105, NO. 4, APRIL 2005. Susan R. Johnson, MD, et. al.

### 47. Effects of Ultra–Low-Dose Transdermal Estradiol on Cognition and Health-Related Quality of Life

Conclusion: Postmenopausal treatment with ultra–low- dose unopposed transdermal estradiol* for 2 years had no effect on change in cognitive function or in health- related quality of life over 2 years of treatment.

*patch, delivering 0.014mg/day ≈ 0.5mg transdermal gel

Yaffee, et al. Arch Neurol .2006;63:945-950

### 48. Endogenous Hormone Levels & Breast Density

Mammographic density well-confirmed predictor of breast cancer risk.

Whether mammographic density reflects levels of endogenous sex hormones is unclear.

Endogenous Hormone Levels, Mammographic Density, and Subsequent Risk of Breast Cancer in Postmenopausal Women

Rulla M. Tamimi, Celia Byrne, Graham A. Colditz, Susan E. J Natl Cancer Inst 2007;99:1178–87

### 49. Estrogen Rx & Breast Density

The study population comprised 158 women: a total of 52 women were using continuous combined HRT (conjugated equine estrogen 0.625 mg plus medroxyprogesterone acetate 5 mg); 51 women were using low-dose oral estrogen alone (estriol 2 mg daily); and 55 women were using unopposed transdermal estrogen given as a patch (estradiol 50 μg/24 h)... An increase in mammographic density was much more common among women taking continuous combined HRT (40%) than for those using oral low-dose estrogen (6%) and transdermal (2%) treatment. ...

E. Lundström, B. Wilczek, Mammographic breast density during hormone replacement therapy: effects of continuous combination, unopposed transdermal and low-potency estrogen regimens et al. Climacteric 2001, Vol. 4, No. 1 , Pages 42-48

### 50. Stroke Risk: TD (Patch) vs Oral

also, Dose Related

The risk of stroke was not increased with use of low oestrogen dose patches [<50mcg] (rate ratio 0.81(0.62 to 1.05)) compared with no use, whereas the risk was increased with high dose patches [>50mcg] (rate ratio 1.89 (1.15 to 3.11)). Current users of oral HRT had a higher rate of stroke than non-users (rate ratio 1.28 (1.15 to 1.42)) with both low dose and high dose.[n = 15710 stroke cases] Transdermal and oral hormone replacement therapy and the risk of stroke: a nested case-control study

BMJ. 2010 Jun 3;340:c2519. doi: 10.1136/bmj.c2519.

### 51. Stroke Risk: Revisited

Conclusions After 10 years of randomised treatment, women receiving hormone replacement therapy early after menopause had a significantly reduced risk of mortality, heart failure, or myocardial infarction, without any apparent increase in risk of cancer, venous thromboembolism, or stroke.[The women in the treated group with an intact uterus started treatment with 2 mg synthetic 17-β-estradiol for 12 days, 2 mg 17-β-estradiol plus 1 mg norethisterone acetate for 10 days, and 1 mg 17-β-estradiol for six days. In women who had undergone hysterectomy, first line treatment was 2 mg 17-β-estradiol a day]

Effect of hormone replacement therapy on cardiovascular events in recently postmenopausal women: randomised trial. BMJ 2012; 345 doi: http://dx.doi.org/10.1136/bmj.e6409 Louise Lind Schierbeck, Lars Rejnmark, et.al.

### 52. Bio-identical Hormones: What's Fact and What's Fable?

The medical literature has established that one of the biggest risk factors for breast cancer is incessant ovulation, that is, ovulating 12 to 13 times per year for 25 to 30 years without any breaks for pregnancy or lactation. Mammary epithelial proliferation occurs with each cycle, causing breast hypertrophy prior to menstruation and a resolution once bleeding occurs. Proliferating breast cells differ from cancer cells only in that they are programmed to stop proliferating at the end of each cycle. In contrast, cancer cells have mutated and lost this control. Therefore, the more menstrual cycles a woman experiences over her lifetime, the greater the risk that a normal proliferating cell will mutate and go on to become a cancer that is not found until 10 to 15 years later.

For postmenopausal women, and especially women who are at higher risk of breast cancer, mimicking "normal" cycles postmenopausally presents the same hormonal environment as incessant ovulation. This is more likely to increase rather than decrease breast cancer risk.

Alan M. Altman, MD, Assistant Clinical Professor, Obstetrics, Gynecology and Reproductive Biology, Harvard Medical School, Boston Mass, srm, Reproduction, & Menopause, April 2007

### 53. Morphological Criteria for the Assessment of Breast Cellular Changes during a Menstrual Cycle

Rathi Ramakrishnan M.D. et. Al.
Mod Pathol 2002;15(12):1348–1356
Morphological Changes in Breast Tissue with Menstrual Cycle

### 54. Dermal Absorption Fatigue

Over several years time, many women using transdermal estrogen preparations have progressively lower urinary estrogens. Sometimes these lower levels are reflected in symptoms, but sometimes (particularly in women who've used bio-identical hormone replacement for longer periods of time) there are no symptoms of these lower estrogen levels. When the route of administration is then switched to intra-vaginal, with no change in dosage, the urinary levels rise once again to the target range, and any symptoms present of low estrogens disappear. We've termed this phenomenon dermal absorption fatigue. As it occurs often, we've switched our routine recommendation for site of bio-identical hormone administration to the intra-vaginal route.

Selected Observations from 23 Years of Bio-Identical Steroid Hormone Replacement in Clinical and Laboratory Practice by Jonathan V. Wright M.D.
Ann N Y Acad Sci. 2005 Dec;1057:506-24

### 55. Progesterone Sensitizes Estrogen Receptors

[Taken From a transcript of a Seminar by Dr John R. Lee, M.D.]    One of the most important lessons I learned. When I give this to a woman who's doctor has her on estrogen, it turns out the dose he has ordered is ALWAYS, two, four, eight, times too much. And I was trying to Figure out, is the doctor that dumb? What is happening here? Why is it that when I give progesterone they get estrogen side effects? They get breast swelling, they get water retention, they get headaches, their feet swell, that's estrogen. Well, it dawned on me finally when I looked it up. Turns out when you have the same hormone all the time like estrogen, unopposed by progesterone, the estrogen receptors tune down. Just as if you're working in an office where there's too much noise. After working there for six months you end up not noticing the noise. Then you go away for two weeks and come back and say, "oh my God, how could I have been working here without realizing all this noise is here?" Every cell that they work on, it does so because there's a receptor, already made that binds and unites with that hormone's molecule, and goes to the nucleus and creates the effects of the message. But it takes binding with that receptor. When you have unopposed estrogen, the receptors tune down. When you add the progesterone the receptors come back to full force again, full efficiency. So, I learned that every time I added progesterone to a woman already on estrogen I had to tell her to cut her

estrogen at least in half. Then later she could cut it down even more because the progesterone was handling so many of her problems. She didn't need all that much estrogen. Then I had some ladies who kept cutting it down, cutting it down and pretty soon they weren't taking any, and they were doing fine. No hot flashes, no vaginal dryness, no problems, they were doing fine and I said, "how can this be?" I was taught in medical school estrogen goes to zero.
http://www.yourlifesource.com/estrogen-receptors.htm

### 56. Transdermal progesterone cream as an alternative to progestin in hormone therapy [effect on endometrial Bx]

Objective: To evaluate the endometrial effects and determine patients' acceptance of transdermal progresterone cream compared to standard hormone therapy.

Methods: Healthy menopausal women received a pretreatment endometrial biopsy (EMB). They were randomized to 0.625 mg conjugated equine estrogen (CEE) daily and 2.5 mg medroxyprogesterone acetate (MPA) (Prempro, Wyeth USA) or daily 0.625 mg CEE and twice daily 20 mg transdermal PC (Pro-gest, Transitions for Health USA). At the end of 6 months, a repeat EMB was obtained, and the women were crossed over to other treatment. A final EMB was performed after the final 6 months.

Results: Twenty-six women completed both arms of the study. 77% of women preferred the CEE/PC to the CEE/MPA (P<.001). Of the 52 post-treatment endometrial biopsies: 40 revealed atrophic endometrium and 12 proliferative endometrium (7 in the oral progestin group and 5 in the PC group). There was no evidence of endometrial hyperplasia in any of the specimens. The incidence of vaginal spotting was similar in both groups.

Conclusion: Patients preferred transdermal PC over oral MPA. This preliminary data indicate that CEE/PC has a similar effect on the endometrium as standard oral HT over a 6-month period.

Leonetti Hb, et al, Altern Ther Health Med. 2005 Nov-Dec;11(6):36-8.

### 57. Comparison of hormone levels in nipple aspirate fluid [NAF] of pre- and postmenopausal women: effect of oral contraceptives and hormone replacement.

Compared with premenopausal women, NAF progesterone was much lower in postmenopausal women...NAF estradiol and estrone sulfate were not significantly less than those in premenopausal women,

...It is concluded that: 1) potential precursors of estradiol remain at comparable levels in the breast after menopause;

Chatterton RT Jr, Geiger AS, Mateo ET, Helenowski IB, Gann PH. J Clin Endocrinol Metab. 2005 Mar;90(3):1686-91.

(Note: Estradiol levels in postmenopausal breast tissue identical to premeno-

pausal breast, yet progesterone much lower. If progesterone protects against breast CA as other evidence suggests, this intra-mammary estrogen dominance would explain increase incidence of breast CA with menopause-HHL)
Hormone Restoration.com Henry Lindner MD
http://hormonerestoration.com/Evidence.html

### 58. Influences of percutaneous administration of estradiol and progesterone on the human breast epithelial cell in vivo.

Objective: To study the effect of E2 and P on the epithelial cell cycle of normal human breast in vivo. DESIGN: Double-blind, randomized study. Topical application to the breast of a gel containing either a placebo, E2, P, or a combination of E2 and P, daily, during the 10 to 13 days preceding breast surgery. PATIENTS: Forty premenopausal women undergoing breast surgery for the removal of a lump. MAIN OUTCOME MEASURES. Plasma and breast tissue concentrations of E2 and P. Epithelial cell cycle evaluated in normal breast tissue areas by counting mitoses and proliferating cell nuclear antigen immunostaining quantitative analyses. RESULTS: Increased E2 concentration increases the number of cycling epithelial cells. Increased P concentration significantly decreases the number of cycling epithelial cells.
Conclusion: Exposure to P for 10 to 13 days reduces E2-induced proliferation of normal breast epithelial cells in vivo.
Chang KJ, Lee TTY et al. Fertil Steril 1995;63:785-91
Hormone Restoration.com Henry Lindner MD
http://hormonerestoration.com/Evidence.html

### 59. Progesterone and Bone: Actions Promoting Bone Health in Women

Abstract
Estradiol (E2) and progesterone (P4) collaborate within bone remodelling on resorption (E2) and formation (P4). We integrate evidence that P4 may prevent and, with antiresorptives, treat women's osteoporosis. P4 stimulates osteoblast differentiation in vitro. Menarche (E2) and onset of ovulation (P4) both contribute to peak BMD. Meta-analysis of 5 studies confirms that regularly cycling premenopausal women lose bone mineral density (BMD) related to subclinical ovulatory disturbances (SODs). Cyclic progestin prevents bone loss in healthy premenopausal women with amenorrhea or SOD. BMD loss is more rapid in perimenopause than postmenopause—decreased bone formation due to P4 deficiency contributes. In 4 placebo-controlled RCTs, BMD loss is not prevented by P4 in postmenopausal women with increased bone turnover. However, 5 studies of E2-MPA co-therapy show greater BMD increases versus E2 alone. P4 fracture data are lacking. P4 prevents bone loss in pre- and possibly perimenopausal women; progesterone co-therapy with anti-resorptives may in-

crease bone formation and BMD.
Journal of Osteoporosis. 2010; 845180.
Vanadin Seifert-Klauss, and Jerilynn C. Prior.
http://www.ncbi.nlm.nih.gov/pmc/articles/PMC2968416/

### 60. Cardiovascular and cancer safety of testosterone in women.

Davis SR.

Purpose of Review:

To examine the recent data pertaining to the relationships between testosterone and cardiovascular disease (CVD) and cancer in women.

Recent Findings:

Despite the entrenched belief that higher blood levels of testosterone increase the risk of CVD in women, data from recent observational studies mostly show an inverse relationship between testosterone and CVD risk. One pilot study suggests favorable effects of nonoral testosterone treatment of women with established congestive cardiac failure which merits further evaluation. The relationship between endogenous testosterone production and breast cancer risk remains contentious, with recent studies indicating either no relationship, or a possible increase in risk when estrone and estradiol are not taken into account. No randomized controlled trial of testosterone therapy has been sufficiently large or of sufficient duration to establish whether such treatment may influence breast cancer occurrence. There does not appear to be an association between testosterone and endometrial cancer, or other malignancies on review of published studies.

Summary: Testosterone is inversely associated with increased CVD risk in women, whereas low sex hormone binding globulin increases CVD risk. The relationship between testosterone and breast cancer remains unclear, although a clear signal of risk has not emerged from studies of women treated with testosterone therapy over the past decade.

Curr Opin Endocrinol Diabetes Obes. 2011 Jun;18(3):198-203. doi: 10.1097/MED.0b013e328344f449.

### 61. Circulating sex steroids and breast cancer risk in premenopausal women.

Recently, the associations between circulating hormones in premenopausal women and subsequent risk of breast cancer have been evaluated. To date, both positive and null associations have been observed for estrogens and inverse and null associations for progesterone with breast cancer risk. For estrogens, the relationships may vary by menstrual cycle phase (e.g., follicular versus luteal phase), although this requires confirmation. Few studies have evaluated estrogen metabolites in relation to breast cancer risk; hence, no conclusions can yet be drawn. Findings for the largely adrenal-derived dehydroepiandrosterone

(DHEA) and DHEA sulfate also are inconsistent and may vary by age. However, relatively consistent positive associations have been observed between testosterone (or free testosterone) levels and breast cancer risk; these associations are of similar magnitude to those confirmed among postmenopausal women. In this review, we summarize current evidence and identify gaps and inconsistencies that need to be addressed in future studies of sex steroids and premenopausal breast cancer risk. Horm Cancer. 2010 Feb;1(1):2-10. doi: 10.1007/s12672-009-0003-0. Epub 2010 Feb 9.
Source
Channing Laboratory, Department of Medicine, Harvard Medical School and Brigham and Women's Hospital,

**62. Associations between serum testosterone levels, cell proliferation and progesterone receptor content in normal and malignant breast tissue in postmenopausal women.**

Progestogens and progesterone receptors (PR) may play an important role in increased breast proliferation following combined estrogen/progestogen hormone therapy, while androgens may counteract this effect. In 50 untreated healthy postmenopausal women and 48 untreated postmenopausal breast cancer patients, we measured serum levels of testosterone (T), sex hormone-binding globulin (SHBG), estrone (E1) and adrenal androgens; and additionally, in the breast cancer patients, cortisol and corticosteroid-binding globulin and endocrine data related to breast proliferation (assessed using the Ki-67/MIB-1 monoclonal antibody) and PR levels (determined by enzyme immunoassay) in the breast cancer tissue. In the healthy women the percentage of MIB-1+ cells showed significant negative correlations with serum levels of total T, calculated free T (fT) and the fT/E1 ratio; while in the breast cancer patients PR content showed significant negative correlations with fT level, the fT/E1 ratio and the T/SHBG ratio. No other correlations were found in any of the groups. Our findings in healthy women confirm previous reports of an antiproliferative effect of androgens in breast tissue and our finding in breast cancer patients suggests that this antiproliferative effect may be mediated via downregulation of PR.
Marie Hofling, Lars Löfgren, et.al.   Gynecological Endocrinology 2008, Vol. 24, No. 7 , Pages 405-410   http://informahealthcare.com/doi/abs/10.1080/09513590802193061

**63. Circulating sex steroids and breast cancer risk in premenopausal women.**
Recently, the associations between circulating hormones in premenopausal women and subsequent risk of breast cancer have been evaluated. To date, both positive and null associations have been observed for estrogens and inverse and null associations for progesterone with breast cancer risk. For estrogens,

the relationships may vary by menstrual cycle phase (e.g., follicular versus luteal phase), although this requires confirmation. Few studies have evaluated estrogen metabolites in relation to breast cancer risk; hence, no conclusions can yet be drawn. Findings for the largely adrenal-derived dehydroepiandrosterone (DHEA) and DHEA sulfate also are inconsistent and may vary by age. However, relatively consistent positive associations have been observed between testosterone (or free testosterone) levels and breast cancer risk; these associations are of similar magnitude to those confirmed among postmenopausal women. In this review, we summarize current evidence and identify gaps and inconsistencies that need to be addressed in future studies of sex steroids and premenopausal breast cancer risk. Horm Cancer. 2010 Feb;1(1):2-10. doi: 10.1007/s12672-009-0003-0. Epub 2010 Feb 9.
Source. Susan E. Hankinson & A. Heather Eliassen
Channing Laboratory, Department of Medicine, Harvard Medical School and Brigham and Women's Hospital.

### 64. Megadose Iodine: An Idea Whose Time Has Come and Gone.

"iodine is a known poison when administered in high doses...."
"Typically the amount of iodine being ingested [12.5-50mg] is 80-300x the RDA and 10-45 x higher than the Tolerable Upper Intake..."
[RDA 150mcg, The Tolerable Upper Intake Level (UL) for adults is 1,100 µg/day (1.1 mg/day)... TUL was assessed by analysing the effect of supplementation on TSH. The thyroid gland needs no more than 70mcg/d to synthesize the requisite amounts of T4 & T3]
"...In Lieu of any credible evidence that high-dose iodine is beneficial (other than for patients with fibrocystic breast changes or a few other clinical conditions), routine use of high-dose iodine should cease..."
Alan Gaby M.D., Editorial Townsend Letter, 12/2010 p 98

### 65. Thyroid: Interesting Facts.

80% of thyroid hormone produced is T4, 20% T3, the more potent form
The bulk [80%] of the T3 your body needs is produced by the conversion of T4 into T3 in the cells of the body, such as liver, kidneys & muscles
"In bloodstream, most of T3 & T4 is bound to TBG* [preferred],
Transthyretin and Albumin. 0.04% T4 and 0.4% of T3 & is free and active!"
T3 has a shorter half-life than T4. T4 remains in the body a lot longer than T3.
Pigs have a higher amount of T3 than humans.
Thyroid Hormone by Theodore C. Friedman, M.D., Ph.D. and Winnie Yu
http://www.thyroid-info.com/articles/hypothyroidism.htm

### 66. Subclinical thyroid disease: scientific review and guidelines for diagnosis and management.

Context: Patients with serum thyroid-stimulating hormone (TSH) levels outside the reference range and levels of free thyroxine (FT4) and triiodothyronine (T3) within the reference range are common in clinical practice. The necessity for further evaluation, possible treatment, and the urgency of treatment have not been clearly established.

Study Selection and Data Extraction: A total of 195 English-language or translated papers were reviewed. Editorials, individual case studies, studies enrolling fewer than 10 patients, and nonsystematic reviews were excluded. Information related to authorship, year of publication, number of subjects, study design, and results were extracted and formed the basis for an evidence report, consisting of tables and summaries of each subject area.

Conclusions: Data supporting associations of subclinical thyroid disease with symptoms or adverse clinical outcomes or benefits of treatment are few. The consequences of subclinical thyroid disease (serum TSH 0.1-0.45 mIU/L or 4.5-10.0 mIU/L) are minimal and we recommend against routine treatment of patients with TSH levels in these ranges. There is insufficient evidence to support population-based screening. Aggressive case finding is appropriate in pregnant women, women older than 60 years, and others at high risk for thyroid dysfunction.

JAMA. 2004 Jan 14;291(2):228-38.Surks MI, et al.

### 67. The Colorado thyroid disease prevalence study.

Participants in a statewide health fair in Colorado, 1995 (N = 25,862).

Results:The prevalence of elevated TSH levels (normal range, 0.3-5.1 mIU/L) in this population was 9.5%, and the prevalence of decreased TSH levels was 2.2%. Forty percent of patients taking thyroid medications had abnormal TSH levels. Lipid levels increased in a graded fashion as thyroid function declined. Also, the mean total cholesterol and low-density lipoprotein cholesterol levels of subjects with TSH values between 5.1 and 10 mIU/L were significantly greater than the corresponding mean lipid levels in euthyroid subjects. Symptoms were reported more often in hypothyroid vs euthyroid individuals, but individual symptom sensitivities were low.

Conclusions:The prevalence of abnormal biochemical thyroid function reported here is substantial and confirms previous reports in smaller populations. Among patients taking thyroid medication, only 60% were within the normal range of TSH. Modest elevations of TSH corresponded to changes in lipid levels that may affect cardiovascular health. Individual symptoms were not very sensitive, but patients who report multiple thyroid symptoms warrant serum thyroid testing. These results confirm that thyroid dysfunction is common, may often go undetected, and may be associated with adverse health outcomes that

can be avoided by serum TSH measurement.
Arch Intern Med. 2000 Feb 28;160(4):526-34.
Canaris GJ, Manowitz NR, Mayor G, Ridgway EC.

### 68. Sex steroids and the thyroid.
Thyroid hormone is affected by Sex Steroids:
Abstract

Thyroid function is modulated by genetic and environmental causes as well as other illnesses and medications such as gonadal or sex steroids. The latter class of drugs (sex steroids) modulates thyroid function. Gonadal steroids exert their influence on thyroid function primarily by altering the clearance of thyroxine-binding globulin (TBG). While oestrogen administration causes an increase in serum TBG concentration, androgen therapy results in a decrease in this binding protein. These effects of gonadal steroids on TBG clearance and concentration are modulated by the chemical structure of the steroid being used, its dose and the route of administration. Despite the gonadal steroids-induced changes in serum TBG concentrations, subjects with normal thyroid glands maintain clinical and biochemical euthyroidism without changes in their serum free thyroxine (T4) or thyroid-stimulating hormone (TSH) levels. In contrast, the administration of gonadal steroids to patients with thyroid diseases causes significant biochemical and clinical alterations requiring changes in the doses of thyroid medications. Similarly, gonadal steroid therapy might unmask thyroid illness in previously undiagnosed subjects. It would be prudent to assess thyroid function in subjects with thyroid disease 6-8 weeks after gonadal steroid administration or withdrawal.
•*Sex steroids and the thyroid.* Tahboub R, Arafah BM.Best Pract Res Clin Endocrinol Metab. 2009 Dec;23(6):769-80. doi: 10.1016/j.beem.2009.06.005.

### 69. Thyroid hormone receptors and reproduction.
J Reprod Immunol. 2011 Jun;90(1):58-66. doi: 10.1016/j.jri.2011.02.009. Epub 2011 Jun 8.. Dittrich R, Beckmann MW, Oppelt PG, Hoffmann I, Lotz L, Kuwert T, Mueller A.
Abstract

Thyroid disorders have a great impact on fertility in both sexes. Hyperthyroidism and hypothyroidism cause changes in sex hormone-binding globulin (SHBG), prolactin, gonadotropin-releasing hormone, and sex steroid serum levels. In females, thyroid hormones may also have a direct effect on oocytes, because it is known that specific binding sites for thyroxin are found on mouse and human oocytes. There is also an association between thyroid dysfunction in women and morbidity and outcome in pregnancy. In males, hyperthyroidism causes a reduction in sperm motility. The numbers of morphologically abnormal sperm are increased by hypothyroidism. When euthyroidism is restored, both abnormalities improve or normalize. In women, the alterations in fertility caused by thyroid disorders are more complex. Hyper- and hypothyroidism are the main thyroid diseases that have an adverse effect on female reproduction and cause menstrual disturbances--mainly hypomenorrhea and polymenorrhea in hyperthyroidism, and oligomenorrhea in hypothyroidism. In recent studies, it has become evident that it is not only changes in serum levels of SHBG and sex steroids that are responsible for these disorders, but also alterations in the metabolic pathway. Adequate levels of circulating thyroid hormones are of primary importance for normal reproductive function. This review presents an overview of the impact of thyroid disorders on reproduction.

### 70. Hypothyroidism might be related to breast cancer in post-menopausal women.

Abstract

An association between breast cancer and thyroid (autoimmune) diseases or the presence of thyroid peroxidase antibodies (TPOAb; a marker of thyroid autoimmune disease) has been suggested. However, little is known about whether women with thyroid (autoimmune) diseases are at increased risk for developing breast cancer. This cross-sectional and prospective cohort study investigated whether the presence of TPOAb or thyroid dysfunction is related to the presence or development of breast cancer. An unselected cohort of 2,775 women around menopause was screened for the thyroid parameters thyrotropin (TSH), free thyroxine (FT(4)), and TPOAb during 1994. Detailed information on previous or actual thyroid disorders and breast cancer, and on putative factors related to breast cancer and thyroid disorders, was obtained. Clinical thyroid dysfunction was defined by both abnormal FT4 and TSH, and subclinical thyroid dysfunction by abnormal TSH (with normal FT4). A TPOAb concentration >or= 100 U/ml was defined as positive (TPOAb(+)). The study group was linked with the Eindhoven Cancer Registry to detect all women with (in situ) breast cancer (ICD-O code 174) diagnosed between 1958 and 1994. Subsequently, in the prospective study, all women who did not have breast cancer in 1994 (n = 2,738) were followed up to July, 2003, and all new cases of (in situ) breast cancer and all cancer-related deaths were registered. Of the 2,775 women, 278 (10.0%) were TPOAb(+). At the 1994 screening, 37 women (1.3%) had breast cancer. TPOAbs were (independently) related to a current diagnosis of breast cancer (OR = 3.3; 95% CI 1.3-8.5). Of the remaining women, 61 (2.2%) developed breast cancer. New breast cancer was related to: (1) an earlier diagnosis of hypothyroidism (OR = 3.8; 95% CI 1.3-10.9); (2) the use of thyroid medication (OR = 3.2; 95% CI 1.0-10.7); and (3) low FT4 (lowest tenth percentile: OR = 2.3; 95% CI 1.2-4.6). In the first 3 years follow up, the relationship between FT4 and log-TSH was disturbed in women with a new breast cancer diagnosis. The presence of TPOAb was not related to breast

cancer during follow-up. A direct relationship between thyroid autoimmunity and breast cancer is unlikely. Hypothyroidism and low-normal FT4 are related with an increased risk of breast cancer in post-menopausal women. Studies are needed to clarify the origins of this possible association.
Thyroid. 2005 Nov;15(11):1253-9. Kuijpens JL, Nyklíctek I, Louwman MW, Weetman TA, Pop VJ, Coebergh JW.

### 71. Armour® Thyroid

Description: (thyroid tablets, USP)* for oral use is a natural preparation derived from porcine thyroid glands and has a strong, characteristic odor. (T3 liothyronine is approximately four times as potent as T4 levothyroxine on a microgram for microgram basis.) They provide 38 mcg levothyroxine (T4) and 9 mcg liothyronine (T3) per grain of thyroid. The inactive ingredients are calcium stearate, dextrose, microcrystalline cellulose, sodium starch glycolate and opadry white.
1 grain of armour provides 38mcg of T4 + 9mcg T3
1.5 grains: 57mcg T4 + 13.5mcg T3
http://www.armourthyroid.com


### 72. Synthroid ingredients:

Active: Synthetic crystalline L-3,3',5,5'-tetraiodothyronine sodium salt with the molecular formula $C1\_(5)H\_(10)I\_(4)N\ NaO\_(4)*H\_(2)O$. Yeah cringe blot it out.. run away!

Inactive: Acacia, confectioner's sugar (contains corn starch), lactose monohydrate, magnesium stearate, povidone, concentration varied food coloring, and talc.

Levoxyl:

Active: synthetic crystalline L-3,3',5,5'-tetraiodothyronine sodium salt with the molecular formula $C1\_(5)H\_(10)I\_(4)N\ NaO\_(4)*H\_(2)O$. Well no change here.. so we have to look to the INERT/INACTIVE ingredients.

Inactive: Microcrystalline cellulose, croscarmellose sodium and magnesium stearate.

Levothyroxine (My Generic ingredients):

Active: synthetic crystalline L-3,3',5,5'-tetraiodothyronine sodium salt with the molecular formula $C1\_(5)H\_(10)I\_(4)N\ NaO\_(4)*H\_(2)O$. Well no change here.. so we have to look to the Inert/Inactive ingredients AGAIN.

Inactive: Magnesium Stearate; Microcrystalline Cellulose; Colloidal Silicone Dioxide; Sodium Starch Glycolate.

The main issue with the inert ingredients is allergic reaction. In Synthroid many have been shown to react adversely to povidone and lactose. Milk allergies even mild ones can respond poorly to constant minute traces of lactose.. inspiring bloating and digestive ills. The cellulose in Levoxyl is just a binding agent and shouldn't interfere with things other than rate of absorption. Croscarmellose sodium toxicological properties have not been fully instigated. WOW!

That is straight off an MSDS sheet. *Snort* I like the generic.. doesn't give me lactose issues and all the inert ingredients have been fully toxicologically profiled.


### 73. Effect of Iodine on Thyroid

Dr Gaby challenges:
that the optimal intake is 13.8mg/day
that the iodine loading test is valid
[50mg intake, ? Amt in urine...
if retained, person considered deficient]
12.5 - 50mg per day is 80 – 333x RDA (150mcg/d)
Literature on Japanese intake: error in interpretation.
Dr Gaby estimates intake at 330 to 500mcg per day.
Iodine overdose is problematic: incl hypo & thyroiditis & hyper
Thyroid function should be monitored if Rx > 1mg/day
Alan Gaby M.D. Editorial.Townsend Letter Aug/Sept 2005


### 74. Hormone Cream Transfer to Children, Pets and Partners

Transdermal Transmission?
Notice Issue: FDA ...is reviewing reports of adverse effects from estradiol transdermal spray (Evamist)...Children unintentionally exposed to the drug through skin contact with women may experience premature puberty. Female children may experience nipple swelling and breast development. Male children may experience breast enlargement.
Recommendation: Patients should make sure that children are not exposed to estradiol transdermal spray and that children do not come into contact with any skin area where the drug was applied.
PubMed Health: U.S. National Library of Medicine
http://www.virginiahopkinstestkits.com/hormone_transfer.html


### 75. Evolution to Lower Doses of Postmenopausal Estrogen Therapy

The clinical use of estrogens to treat menopausal symptoms was first described nearly 80 years ago. In the early 1940s oral estrogen formulations for post-menopausal hormonal therapy (HT) became available and, since that time, doses of estrogen in HT have been continually decreasing. Until the mid-1970s daily doses of conjugated equine estrogens (CEE) as high as 1.25 mg or 2.5 mg were commonly used, thereafter transitioning to 0.625 mg/day as the standard dose. Use of the lowest clinically effective dose of HT for relief of menopause-related symptoms and for prevention of osteoporosis is now rec-ommended. Low-dose estrogen therapy (ET) is currently defined as a dose of

oral CEE of ≤0.45 mg/d, oral estradiol ≤0.5 mg/d, transdermal estradiol ≤0.025 mg/d. These lower doses of estrogen are increasingly being recommended for relief of menopausal symptoms, as well as for prevention of osteoporosis in post-menopausal women. Michelle P. Warren, MD Dec. 2008
Other writing by Michelle Warren MD in Endotext:
https://www.ncbi.nlm.nih.gov/books/NBK279050/

### 76. HRT in older women: Is it ever too late?

BCMJ, Vol. 43, No. 9, November 2001, page(s) 517-521. Margo R. Fluker, MD, FRCSC

For many mature women and their health care providers, the initial discussion about the risks and benefits of hormone replacement therapy occurs around the time of the menopause and is triggered by the onset of vasomotor symptoms. However, the opportunity for a second discussion about HRT may arise again in the seventh decade or beyond, and is often triggered by an adverse health event in the woman or someone close to her. The latter opportunity should not be overlooked, as it provides a chance to re-evaluate various lifestyle factors, concomitant medication use, musculoskeletal health, cardiac health, and uro-genital/sexual health.

If the risk-benefit ratio favors HRT, various strategies can be used to improve acceptance and minimize side effects. These include instituting therapy slowly, considering lower doses, and evaluating systemic versus local therapy. While there are many inevitable health consequences of menopause and aging, the initiation of systemic or local HRT may be both appropriate and acceptable in some older women in order to improve the quality, if not the quantity, of life.

### 77. Estrogen and Coagulation

Double blind, randomized study of estradiol replacement therapy on markers of inflammation, coagulation and fibrinolysis.
Atherosclerosis, 2003, vol. 168, no1, pp. 123-129. Zegura B, Keber I, Sebestjen M, Koenig W. There was no influence of transdermal E2 on markers of coagulation activation, fibrinolysis and inflammation, but it decreased fibrinogen levels significantly.

### 78. Effects of oral and transdermal estrogen/progesterone regimens on blood coagulation and fibrinolysis in postmenopausal women. A randomized controlled trial.

We conclude that oral estrogen/progesterone replacement therapy may result in coagulation activation and increased fibrinolytic potential, whereas opposed transdermal estrogen appears without any substantial effects on hemostasis.
Arterioscler Thromb Vasc Biol. 1997 Nov;17(11):3071-8. Scarabin PY, Alhenc-Gelas M, Plu-Bureau G, Taisne P, Agher R, Aiach M.

**79. Reduced Estriol Excretion in Patients With Breast Cancer Prior to Endocrine Therapy** JAMA. 1966;196(13):1128-1136. Henry M. Lemon, MD; Herbert H. Wotiz, PhD; Langdon Parsons, MD; Peter J. Mozden, MD

**80. Reducing the Hormone Related Cancer Risk (Or cabbages, sex hormones and their metabolites).** Jonathan Wright MD Nutrition and Healing (USA 800 528 0559) ,
https://www.antiaging-systems.com/articles/129-cancer-risk-reduction
One of the first theories about estrogen and cancer was advanced by Henry Lemon, M.D. of the University of Nebraska. Focusing on estriol (the principal circulating estrogen), Dr. Lemon initially argued that greater proportions of estriol are good, and perhaps even anti-carcinogenic. He found that women most likely to survive breast cancer had the largest amounts of estriol. In unpublished work on a small, uncontrolled study, estriol administration appeared to cause remission in a proportion of breast cancers that had metastasized to bone.
Other researchers discovered that Asian women living in Asia, who as a group have lower rates of breast cancer, also had higher proportions of circulating estriol than American women, who have higher rates of breast cancer. Asian women living in Hawaii, who have a breast cancer rate midway between Asian women living in Asia and American women, also have estriol levels midway between those of the other two groups. Sisters and daughters of women who had had breast cancer were found to have lower proportions of estriol than sisters and daughters of women without breast cancer. Considerable animal research appeared to indicate that estriol was anti-carcinogenic or at least non-carcinogenic. However, other research20 disputed the "estriol hypothesis", and present-day researchers tend to disregard it in favor of other theories.

**81. Estriol: Its Weakness is Its Strength**
By Olivia A.M. Franks, ND and Jonathan V. Wright, MD, Life Extension Scientific Advisory Board Member
What you need to know:
The body naturally makes three estrogen hormones—estradiol, estrone, and estriol. Since estriol possesses the weakest estrogenic effects of the three, it has been largely overlooked by the medical community.
Many studies show that estriol offers a wealth of potential health benefits—without the dangers that sometimes accompany higher-potency estrogens and synthetic or horse-derived hormones.
Studies suggest that estriol helps relieve menopausal symptoms while benefitting bone and urinary tract health. Estriol may also help improve cardiovascular risk factors and even shows promise in reducing the brain lesions of multiple sclerosis.
The most reliable way to measure estriol levels is through 24-hour urine collection.

Despite abundant evidence to the contrary, the FDA has recently claimed that estriol is not safe. You can act now to help preserve consumers' access to bi-oidentical hormones such as estriol by visiting www.homecoalition.org.

Fear of cancer prevents many women from restoring youthful hormone levels. When applied through the topical (transdermal) route, estriol is not associated with increased cancer risk. Other methods women can use to prevent hormone-related cancers include consuming abundant vitamin D, cruciferous vegetables, soy, D-glucarate, and lignans, while minimizing meat and high-fat dairy intake.

Life Extension: http://www.lifeextension.com/magazine/2008/8/estriol-its-weakness-is-its-strength/page-01

### 82. Are Transdermals Transmitted to Spouse and Others by Contact?

We sampled the thigh skin of a 54 year old woman who had been applying transdermal E2 daily. The first samples were taken prior to hormone application Then a total of 2mg E2 was applied to a section of both thighs.

Application locations were divided into sectors.

Swabs were taken of a sector at different post application times

Each swab sampled a sector that contained $0.25mg = 250\mu g$ E2

Swabs were analyzed for E2 content by Rhein Labs, Portland Oregon, Frank Nordt PhD, director.

Skin levels prior to application, after shower: 0.04mcg. 3 minutes after application of estradiol to skin: 17mcg. 2 hours after application: 4.7mcg. 3 minutes after thorough washing of site of application: 0.06mcg.

### 83. Eating behavior and adherence to dietary prescriptions in obese adult subjects treated with 5-hydroxytryptophan.

Am J Clin Nutr. 1992 Nov;56(5):863-7.

Cangiano C1, Ceci F, Cascino A, Del Ben M, Laviano A, Muscaritoli M, Antonucci F, Rossi-Fanelli F.

Author information   https://www.ncbi.nlm.nih.gov/pubmed/1384305

Abstract

Previous observations have shown that oral administration of 5-hydroxytryptophan (5-HTP) without dietary prescriptions causes anorexia, decreased food intake, and weight loss in obese subjects. To confirm these data over a longer period of observation and to verify whether adherence to dietary restriction could be improved by 5-HTP, 20 obese patients were randomly assigned to receive either 5-HTP (900 mg/d) or a placebo. The study was double-blinded and was for two consecutive 6-wk periods. No diet was prescribed during the first period, a 5040-kJ/d diet was recommended for the second. Significant weight loss was observed in 5-HTP-treated patients during both periods. A reduction in carbohydrate intake and a consistent presence of early satiety were also found. These findings together with the good tolerance observed suggest that 5-HTP may be safely used to treat obesity.

### 84. Effects of oral 5-hydroxy-tryptophan on energy intake and macronutrient selection in non-insulin dependent diabetic patients.

https://www.ncbi.nlm.nih.gov/pubmed/9705024
Int J Obes Relat Metab Disord. 1998 Jul;22(7):648-54.
Cangiano Cl, Laviano A, Del Ben M, Preziosa I, Angelico F, Cascino A, Rossi-Fanelli F. Author information     https://www.ncbi.nlm.nih.gov/pubmed/9705024

Abstract
Objective:
In obese patients, brain serotonergic stimulation via orally administered 5-hydroxy-tryptophan (5-HTP), the precursor of serotonin, causes decreased carbohydrate intake and weight loss. Since diabetes mellitus is associated with depressed brain serotonin, hyperphagia and carbohydrate craving, we hypothesized that in diabetic patients, orally administered 5-HTP stimulates brain serotonergic activity and thus normalizes eating behaviour. To test this hypothesis, we investigated whether in diabetic patients: 1) predicted brain serotonin concentrations are depressed as a result of decreased availability of the precursor, tryptophan; and 2) oral 5-HTP is effective in reducing energy and carbohydrate intake.

Subjects and Methods: 25 Overweight non-insulin dependent diabetic outpatients were enrolled in a double-blind, placebo-controlled study, and randomized to receive either 5-HTP (750 mg/d) or placebo for two consecutive weeks, during which no dietary restriction was prescribed.

Methods:
Energy intake and eating behaviour, as expressed by macronutrient selection, were evaluated using a daily diet diary. Plasma amino acid concentrations and body weight, as well as serum glucose, insulin and glycosylated haemoglobin were assessed.

Results:
20 patients (nine from the 5-HTP group and 11 from the Placebo group) completed the study. Brain tryptophan availability in diabetic patients was significantly reduced when compared to a group of healthy controls. Patients receiving 5-HTP significantly decreased their daily energy intake, by reducing carbohydrate and fat intake, and reduced their body weight.

Conclusions:
These data confirm the role of the serotonergic system in reducing energy intake, by predominantly inhibiting carbohydrate intake, and suggest that 5-HTP may be safely utilized to improve the compliance to dietary prescriptions in non-insulin dependent diabetes mellitus.

### 85. 5-Hydroxytryptophan: a clinically-effective serotonin precursor.

Altern Med Rev. 1998 Aug;3(4):271-80.

Birdsall TC1.

Author information   https://www.ncbi.nlm.nih.gov/pubmed/9727088

Abstract

5-Hydroxytryptophan (5-HTP) is the intermediate metabolite of the essential amino acid L-tryptophan (LT) in the biosynthesis of serotonin. Intestinal absorption of 5-HTP does not require the presence of a transport molecule, and is not affected by the presence of other amino acids; therefore it may be taken with meals without reducing its effectiveness. Unlike LT, 5-HTP cannot be shunted into niacin or protein production. Therapeutic use of 5-HTP bypasses the conversion of LT into 5-HTP by the enzyme tryptophan hydroxylase, which is the rate-limiting step in the synthesis of serotonin. 5-HTP is well absorbed from an oral dose, with about 70 percent ending up in the bloodstream. It easily crosses the blood-brain barrier and effectively increases central nervous system (CNS) synthesis of serotonin. In the CNS, serotonin levels have been implicated in the regulation of sleep, depression, anxiety, aggression, appetite, temperature, sexual behaviour, and pain sensation. Therapeutic administration of 5-HTP has been shown to be effective in treating a wide variety of conditions, including depression, fibromyalgia, binge eating associated with obesity, chronic headaches, and insomnia.

### 86. Tyrosine, phenylalanine, and catecholamine synthesis and function in the brain.

Fernstrom JD1, Fernstrom MH.

J Nutr. 2007 Jun;137(6 Suppl 1):1539S-1547S; discussion 1548S.

https://www.ncbi.nlm.nih.gov/pubmed/17513421

Abstract

Aromatic amino acids in the brain function as precursors for the monoamine neurotransmitters serotonin (substrate tryptophan) and the catecholamines [dopamine, norepinephrine, epinephrine; substrate tyrosine (Tyr)]. Unlike almost all other neurotransmitter biosynthetic pathways, the rates of synthesis of serotonin and catecholamines in the brain are sensitive to local substrate concentrations, particularly in the ranges normally found in vivo. As a consequence, physiologic factors that influence brain pools of these amino acids, notably diet, influence their rates of conversion to neurotransmitter products, with functional consequences. This review focuses on Tyr and phenylalanine (Phe). Elevating brain Tyr concentrations stimulates catecholamine production, an effect exclusive to actively firing neurons. Increasing the amount of protein ingested, acutely (single meal) or chronically (intake over several days), raises brain Tyr concentrations and stimulates catecholamine synthesis. Phe, like Tyr, is a substrate for Tyr hydroxylase, the enzyme catalyzing the rate-limiting step in catecholamine synthesis. Tyr is the preferred substrate; consequently, unless Tyr concentrations are abnormally low, variations in Phe concentration do not affect catecholamine synthesis. Unlike Tyr, Phe does not demonstrate substrate inhibition. Hence, high concentrations of Phe do not inhibit catecholamine synthesis and probably are not responsible for the low production of catecholamines in subjects with phenylketonuria. Whereas neuronal catecholamine release varies directly with Tyr-induced changes in catecholamine synthesis, and brain functions linked pharmacologically to catecholamine neurons are predictably altered, the physiologic functions that utilize the link between Tyr supply and catecholamine synthesis/release are presently unknown. An attractive candidate is the passive monitoring of protein intake to influence protein-seeking behavior.

# Index

Here is what I believe are the most important things that you might want to know about menopause and bio-identical hormones:

- Menopause can feel challenging, both with the symptoms that have developed and about the safety of treatment with hormones.

- Many women who have received good treatment have succeeded in feeling better. Most importantly, in the process of being treated, they have done so much toward preventing the deeper issues that result over time from low ovarian hormones, which can affect the rest of their lives.

  o Thus, symptom alleviation of hot flashes, sleep disturbance, cognitive decline, skin and hair changes, mood deterioration, libido decline, energy loss, etc. is so important and rewarding.

  o From a medical perspective and, most importantly, for a woman's well-being, all that can be achieved in the prevention of osteoporosis, sarcopenia (loss of skeletal muscle and, thus, weakness and instability), blood vessel risk, cognitive issues, bladder disturbances, vaginal atrophy, and more is the most rewarding of all. Older women do not like the bladder problems that lead to the use of adult padded underwear, canes, walkers, and wheel chairs, not to mention the fractures and the equalization of cardiac risk that occur in men by the age of 60. All of these issues and more can result from not attending to ovarian hormone decline.

- Risk is on every woman's mind. Here is a summary of what I conclude as a medical doctor in practice for 49 years and from the results of extensive scientific medical studies:
  - We are all at risk for serious illnesses, even more so as we grow older, from a multitude of causes that are often cumulative over a lifetime.
  - Breast cancer risk is less for menopausal women who are treated with bio-identical hormones than for those who receive no treatment at all.
- Breast cancers can take 10 to 15 years to develop from one cell all the way to becoming a discoverable cancer. Cancers have many causes. I believe that no hormone causes cancer. However, if a breast cancer is non-primitive—"well-differentiated"—it looks and behaves like a normal breast glandular cell. If it has estrogen receptor sites (as a normal breast cell does), it will tend to grow more rapidly in a premenopausal woman who still has her natural and robust estrogen hormones present. If you treat a menopausal woman who has this type of cancer already present, it will tend to grow faster than if she was not treated with hormones.
- There is no place for treating women in menopause with youthful levels of ovarian hormones.
- Lowish dosages (precisely defined in our professional training program) work well in achieving symptom alleviation and providing protection to crucial organs.
- Based on my conclusions from the medical literature, excessive dosages are definitely not called for; they can cause breast glandular proliferation, consequently increasing breast density and, thus, increasing risk!

- On the other hand, there is medical research evidence that proper treatment with ovarian hormones provides significant protection to the bones, muscles, arteries, brain, vagina, bladder, and more.

- Individuality prevails in treating women in menopause with hormones. Women vary as to how much of each hormone they need; how well they can absorb it from their skin; how sensitive they are to what they absorb, and how they respond, etc. For these reasons, dosages are best determined by each individual woman, beginning with guidelines from her physician or nurse practitioner and through a process of "titration." Treatment begins with low dosages that are gradually increased until symptoms of hormonal insufficiency (such as hot flashes) are alleviated. At the same time, we fall shy of or back down from symptoms of hormonal excess (such as breast tenderness), which could occur if dosages get too high.

- There are many hormone choices available on the market. Once you learn about the details of "bio-identical" hormones—those that are molecularly identical to the hormones once produced by your ovaries—I believe you will want no other type!

- For maximum safety:

  - Estrogens and testosterone should only be administered by transdermal or transmucosal application. They should not be taken by mouth.

  - Progesterone and DHEA are best administered by transdermal or transmucosal routes. If adequate dosages cannot be achieved through these routes, oral administration is fine for either or both of these two hormones.

- The best of the bio-identical hormones available are being prepared by "compounding" pharmacists in your own community. They procure FDA chemically-pure hormones from pharmaceutical manufacturers who extract the hormones with great precision from plants. The pharmacists then add the hormones to "bases," so you can apply them to your skin or mucous membranes. Those bases are most commonly strong solvents. They need to be strong because hormones are not dissolvable in water; they are only (and poorly) soluble in solvents capable of dissolving fats. Because these strong solvents may have toxic potential, even if ever so slight, I recommend that your compounding pharmacist purchase and use the organic, non-solvent base to formulate the hormones for administration. These hormones will not be in a solution, so the bottle will need to be shaken before each use. (For further information, your pharmacist can go to www.menopausemethod.com, and select "For Pharmacists.")

- Gone are the days of "one or two pills fit all." Over the last 30 years, the knowledge and experience base of treating women in menopause with bio-identical hormones has mushroomed. e.g., I recommend that every woman seek assistance from a medical professional (physician, nurse practitioner or, in states that approve, prescribing pharmacist) who has received advanced education in this field. (One source of advanced training is www.menopausemethod.com. Select "For Medical Professionals.")

- Perhaps the most important thing I have to say to you is that 24-hour urine hormone testing is absolutely imperative once you have titrated to what seems to be good symptom relief. At that time, we always test to determine if your hormone levels fall into what are considered to be optimal ranges: not too high and not too low.

o There is absolutely no getting around this! No matter how specifically your medical professional has prescribed what seems to be safe dosages, and no matter how precisely you have titrated to symptom alleviation, these parameters are just not reliable enough to determine if your hormone levels are within the optimal range. Because of differences in absorption, sensitivity, needs, responses, etc., from one woman to the next, it is not possible to predict with enough accuracy whether a woman has achieved optimal hormone levels, or is on too low or too high of a dosage. I have determined this from decades of careful testing. At least 25% of my most symptom-satisfied patients and those who seem to be within the proper dose range for four hormones will test too low or too high. Levels that are too low are not sufficient to protect organs over the long term. At the same time, levels that are too high are a poor choice when working with biochemicals as potent as hormones and, in my opinion, puts women at risk.

• Regarding the androgens, DHEA and testosterone, I almost always prefer to begin treatment of women in menopause with Bi-Est (the estrogens) and progesterone. For optimal health, sooner or later, every woman will also need to be treated with DHEA and testosterone. One of the main—and far from the only—reasons is that whether at the beginning of menopause or within 3 to 4 years maximum, every woman's androgen levels will be lower than optimal to support and protect the muscles, mood, energy, resilience, and more. At the time of their first consultation for menopause, some women are obviously already depleted in androgens, based on clinical signs and symptoms alone. We begin androgens during the second consultation with these women, giving them over a month to get a "sense" of and titrate to optimal levels of Bi-Est and progesterone. If a women is not obviously androgen-depleted initially, we will wait for the results of their first 24-hour urine hormone test to assess their androgen levels accurately. This usually occurs in the 3rd or 4th month of the initial treatment process. In my experience, even if a woman's initial test result reveals reasonable androgen levels, by 2 to 4 years from that time, every woman will be androgen-depleted and, thus, will benefit from treatment.

- Once dosages and balances are reached, and your 24-hour urine hormone test result is evaluated and deemed acceptable, annual follow-up with your healthcare provider is essential. In our program, that annual consultation will include the following:
  - ○ Routine female exams.
  - ○ Testing. The rate of the repetition of the following tests are flexible and depend on the medical circumstances of the individual patient.

Testing includes:

- Appropriate blood tests: annually, to every 2 to 3 years.
- 24-hour urine hormone test: every 1 to 2 years.
- Mammogram: every 1 to 4 years.
- Bone density test: every 1 to 4 years.
- Transvaginal ultrasound for women with a uterus and/ or ovaries: every 1 to 3 years.

- Breast thermography when indicated in women with increased breast density: every 1 to 4 years.

- Treating women in menopause occurs at the 50,000-mile mark of our lives. By this time, there is much water under the bridge, including many adversities of nutrition, exercise (insufficient or excessive), toxic exposure, and the elephant in all of our rooms: an excessive, and thus, health-challenging response to the stress in our lives. So, although much can be achieved with hormones, it is an important time of life to evaluate other possible health issues, apparent or hidden, and address them with as much commitment as absolutely possible! You will want so much to be in good enough health as you age! Just ask anyone who is significantly older than you are! An ounce of prevention is worth a ton of cure.

- How early does one start hormones?

  - The best case is to be on the lookout after age 35 when it is common for progesterone to decline more rapidly than estrogen: these women can definitely benefit from optimal amounts of transdermal progesterone.

  - Beyond that, as early as you possibly can, when the symptoms inspire you to do so or even if you do not have any symptoms at all!

- Is it ever too late to begin? Let me answer this with one word: no.

- How long should one treat? Let me answer this best by saying I started treating my mother and mother-in-law in their late eighties, and much to their benefit.

If your healthcare provider is new to treating women in menopause with bio-identical hormones, yet is open to exploring this field, you will be able to work synergistically with them to develop your program. We are happy to consult with your provider free of charge to assist them in learning and implementing more. In addition, we offer an extensive professional training program: visit www.menopausemethod.com, and select "For Professionals."

Warm regards and best wishes to you,

# Patient Dose Determination Tool: Titration

## Finding Your Optimal Hormone Dose by Alleviating Symptoms of Insufficiency While Falling Shy of or Backing Down from Symptoms of Excess:
### *Estrogens*

---

### Finding Your Optimal Dose

**ESTROGENS**

**Too little:**
- Warm rushes
- Night sweats
- Sleep disturbance*
- Mental fogginess &/or forgetfulness
- Weight gain (primarily thighs, hips &/or buttocks)
- Dry vagina, eyes &/or skin
- Diminished sensuality & sexuality*
- Sense of normalcy only during 2nd week (if cycling)
- Hot flashes*
- Temperature swings
- Racing mind at night
- Fatigue or reduced stamina
- Episodes of rapid heartbeat &/or palpitations
- Pain during intercourse
- Loss of glow
- Back &/or joint pain
- Intestinal bloating
- Headaches &/or migraines

**Too much:**
- Breast tenderness*
- Breast fullness
- Impatient but clear of mind
- Pelvic cramps (w or w/o bleeding)
- Nipple tenderness
- Malaise
- Water retention (swollen fingers, legs &/or ankles)
- Hot flashes* (if excessive dose!)

---

*\* These symptoms can have more than one cause.*
*When in doubt, call your doctor*

***Do not exceed your doctor's suggested maximum dosages***

 For important instructions on how to apply hormones, go to:

---

# Patient Dose Determination Tool: Titration

## Finding Your Optimal Hormone Dose by Alleviating Symptoms of Insufficiency While Falling Shy of or Backing Down from Symptoms of Excess:
### *Progesterone and Testosterone*

**Finding Your Optimal Dose**

### PROGESTERONE

**Too little:**
- Sleep disturbance*
- Increased anxiety
- Mood disturbances
  (sometimes severe)
- Hot flashes*
- Breast tenderness*
- New &/or enlarged breast lumps
- Water retention*
- Difficulty relaxing
- Decreased libido*
- Period irregularities
  (if still menstruating)
- PMS, fibroids, &/or endometriosis

**Too much:**
- Drowsiness
- Waking up groggy &/or edgy
- Sense of physical instability
- Hot flashes* (if very excessive dose!)
- Feeling depressed
- Slight dizziness
- Leg discomfort/pain
- Water retention*

### TESTOSTERONE

**Too little:**
- Diminished libido*
- Loss of sense of security
- Body hair loss
- Diminished energy/stamina
- Flabbiness/muscular weakness
  (upper arms, thighs, & cheeks)

**Too much:**
- Hyper-aggressiveness
- Excessive oiliness of skin
- Increased pimples/acne
- Increased hair growth on body, face, &/or place of application

*\* These symptoms can have more than one cause.
When in doubt, call your doctor*

# About the Author

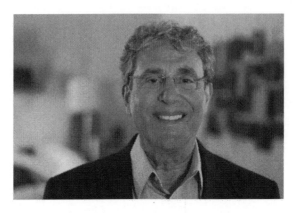

## Daved Rosensweet M.D.

Dr. Rosensweet graduated from the University of Michigan Medical School in 1968. While his knowledge is based on his traditional training, he integrates information and tools learned from renowned pioneers and practitioners in the holistic and healing fields. He has been in private holistic medical practice since 1971 and has had offices in New Mexico, California, Colorado, and Florida. Early in his career, he delivered over 300 babies at home. Dr. Rosensweet trained the first nurse practitioners in the United States, was in charge of health promotion for the State of New Mexico, and was the chief investigator of a hormone study for an American reference laboratory. He lectures widely, teaching menopause medicine to medical professionals in live seminars as well as online at www.menopausemethod.com. He is currently in private practice in Sarasota, Florida and is medical director of www.iwonderdoctor.com.

Printed in Great Britain
by Amazon

57227265R00194